Praise for

"*Be Heart Smart* is a comprehensive analysis of the risk factors, diagnostic evaluation, and treatment of coronary heart disease. It should be read by anyone with a family history of a heart attack or a fear of experiencing one. If everyone in the United States followed the recommendations, tens of thousands of lives would be saved each year."
—**Robert Pearl, MD**, bestselling author of *Mistreated: Why We Think We're Getting Good Health Care and Why We're Usually Wrong*

"Dr. Khan has distilled the complexities of heart disease to make them easily understandable by the layperson—our patients. It is well-written, informative, and fun to read. It offers excellent advice, which reflects the experience and good judgment of the author. I highly recommend this for all patients with heart and vascular problems."
—**Mahesh Ramchandani MD, FRCS**, Chief of Cardiac Surgery at DeBakey Heart and Vascular Center at Houston Methodist Hospital

"Dr. Khan is a terrific writer, and his book on heart health is the best I've read—clear, focused, and friendly. I intend to read it regularly to maintain my heart. I was especially happy to see him point to depression as a problem. As I would put it, the soul, not just the body, can have a heart attack."
—**Thomas Moore**, author of the *New York Times* bestseller *Care of the Soul*

"A writer's most challenging task is to take a complicated, angst-ridden subject, and render it simple and even enjoyable. Dr. Khan has accomplished this feat with the human heart. Consider this book the essential owner's manual for that life-sustaining machine."
—**Jay Heinrichs**, author of the *New York Times* bestseller *Thank You for Arguing*

"*Be Heart Smart* is the practical, pragmatic, down-to-earth book for patients that every cardiology patient should read, and every cardiologist wishes they had written. I'm definitely purchasing copies for my family!"
—**Halee Fischer-Wright, MD**, CEO of the Medical Group Management Association and bestselling author of *Back to Balance*

"Be Heart Smart is written by a very experienced physician who has been diagnosing and treating patients for many years. This book shares real-life experiences that Dr. Khan has had with patients with different forms of coronary artery disease and informs patients about causes, consequences, optimal treatments, and efforts to prevent them. I recommend this book to all patients who have coronary artery disease and for their family and friends."
—**James T. Willerson, MD**, President Emeritus of Texas Heart Institute, former editor of the American Heart Association journal *Circulation*, Past-President of the University of Texas Health Science Center, and author of numerous books, including *Coronary Artery Disease* and *Cardiovascular Medicine*

"Be Heart Smart is easy to read and well-directed at the layman—very comprehensive for the patient concerned about CHD."
—**Morton J. Kern, MD**, Past President of Society for Cardiovascular Angiography and Interventions and author of *The Cardiac Catheterization Handbook*

"This is a practical guide to help individuals understand the signs and symptoms of heart disease and the approach to both treat and prevent heart disease."
—**Christie Ballantyne, MD**, Chief of Cardiology and Cardiovascular Research at Baylor College of Medicine

"Dr. Khan has delivered a valuable read for anyone concerned about heart health. Clear, well organized, and potentially life-saving information is presented in an easy-to-understand format. Well done!"
—**Rick Kirschner, MD**, bestselling author of *How to Deal with Difficult People*

"This excellent book is written with great clarity in a way that a lay readership can gain a better understanding of the protocols for treating and possibly reducing the risk of developing heart disease."
—**Marcus Conyers, PhD**, author of *Positively Smarter: Science and Strategies for Increasing Happiness, Achievement, and Well-Being*

BE HEART SMART

UNDERSTAND, TREAT, AND PREVENT
CORONARY HEART DISEASE

BE HEART
SMART

UNDERSTAND, TREAT, AND PREVENT
CORONARY HEART DISEASE

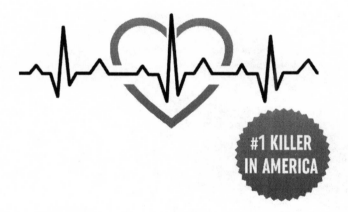

#1 KILLER
IN AMERICA

WAQAR KHAN, MD MPH

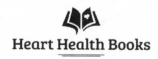

Heart Health Books

SPRING, TEXAS

Disclaimer

Be Heart Smart offers health, fitness, and nutritional information and is for educational purposes only. This book is intended to supplement, not replace, the professional medical advice, diagnosis, or treatment of health conditions from a trained health professional. Please consult your physician or other healthcare professional before beginning or changing any health or fitness program to make sure that it is appropriate for your needs—especially if you are pregnant or have a family history of any medical concerns, illnesses, or risks. If you have any concerns or questions about your health, you should always consult with a physician or other healthcare professional. Stop exercising immediately if you experience faintness, dizziness, pain, or shortness of breath at any time. Please do not disregard, avoid, or delay obtaining medical or health-related advice from your healthcare professional because of something you may have read in this guide.

Heart Health Books
58 Mediterra Way
Spring, TX 77389

For more information, visit www.HeartHealthBooks.com or email hearthealthbooks@gmail.com.

Project Management by Markman Editorial Services: www.MarlaMarkman.com
Book Design by GKS Creative: www.gkscreative.com

Publisher's Cataloging-in Publication data
Names: Khan, Waqar, author.
Titles: Be heart smart : understand , treat and prevent coronary heart disease / Waqar Khan, MD, MPH
Description: Includes index. | Spring, TX: Heart Health Books, 2018.
Identifiers: ISBN 978-1-7322686-0-9 | LCCN 2018905631
Subjects: LCSH Coronary heart disease. | Heart--Diseases--Prevention. | Heart--Popular works. | BISAC HEALTH & FITNESS / Diseases / Heart
Classification: LCC RC682 .K49 2018 | DDC 616.1/205

ISBN: 978-1-7322686-0-9 Print Book
ISBN: 978-1-7322686-1-6 E-Book

Printed in the United States of America

24 23 22 21 20 19 18   10 9 8 7 6 5 4 3 2 1

To my parents: I am who I am because of you.

To my wife: for all your consistent support and for believing in me.

To my children: You are the spice of my life and you make life so much fun.

TABLE OF CONTENTS

INTRODUCTION

*W*hy did this happen to me?
I often hear this question from my patients after they have suffered a heart attack, experienced a frightening episode of chest pain, or been diagnosed with coronary heart disease (CHD). As a board-certified interventional cardiologist in private practice for more than 20 years in suburban Houston, I've heard this question from people of all ages and all walks of life—executives, construction workers, tech industry leaders, teachers, firefighters, pilots, stay-at-home moms, and more.

Countless times in my career, I've told my patients about the causes and risk factors for CHD, which leads to an estimated 735,000 heart attacks per year. And I've filled them in on the latest treatment options and lifestyle changes that can improve their health and help them prevent future heart attacks. But like most busy doctors, I don't always have time to fully explain everything about CHD and the exciting advances in its treatment. That's where this book comes in. I wanted to find a way to give my patients and others detailed information they can use to take charge of their heart health.

This book is intended to offer detailed answers to the questions I hear on a daily basis in my office. You may have many of these same questions. Although primarily intended as a resource for patients with CHD, this book also serves as a guide for family members and friends who are supporting their loved ones through the process. It can also help you gain a better understanding of CHD and discover topics you may want to discuss further with your own doctor to ensure you are doing everything possible to enhance your well-being.

The information in these pages is based on the most up-to-date, rigorous scientific evidence. I hope it will serve as an eye-opener to show you that having a heart attack or getting a diagnosis of CHD isn't the end of your life. Instead, it can be the beginning of a new heart-smart lifestyle that will lower your risk of future coronary events and help keep your heart healthy for years to come.

PART I

UNDERSTANDING CORONARY

HEART DISEASE

"The only lasting beauty is the beauty of the heart."
— Rumi

CHAPTER 1

HEART BASICS: CORONARY HEART DISEASE, ACUTE CORONARY SYNDROME, AND HEART ATTACK

It was a typical Saturday. I was on call at a local hospital in suburban Houston, and since it was a quiet morning, I was catching up on some recent studies in a few medical journals. As an interventional cardiologist, I like to stay on top of the most up-to-date research and cutting-edge techniques that can help my patients. In the middle of reading an article, I got an urgent call to the emergency room. As I arrived, the ER doors swung open and paramedics wheeled in a patient—male, 45, chest pain, unconscious.

We transported him to the cardiac catheterization lab—the cath lab—to run tests to see what was happening with his heart. As we ran the imaging diagnostics, the patient flatlined again as he had done prior to arriving in the ER. We had to shock his heart multiple times to bring him back to life. The images told a worst-case scenario. He had a severe blockage in the most catastrophic spot—an artery cardiologists refer to as the "widowmaker." The left anterior descending artery supplies blood to a large portion of the heart, and when it is blocked, it often results in sudden death.

When I realized the blockage was in the widowmaker, I thought about his wife, who had told me while sobbing in the ER that her husband was an airline pilot. I didn't want her to become a widow that day, but I knew that her husband's chances of survival were slim—few people who suffer a heart attack due to a blockage in the widowmaker make it out of the hospital alive. We immediately put the man on a ventilator and inserted a lifesaving mechanical balloon-pump device to help his heart pump more blood to his coronary arteries while we removed the blockage—a large blood clot—and placed a stent in the artery. With the stent in place, blood resumed flow to his heart, and it started beating normally again. Fortunately, his wife would not become a widow that day.

The following day we removed the ventilator, and when the airline pilot woke up, his chest pain was gone and his electrocardiogram (EKG) showed improvement. His wife was overjoyed to see him doing so much better, and a couple days later, he left the hospital. In time, he resumed his job as a pilot. Now I see him on a regular basis for follow-ups; his heart is healthy, and he feels great. The pilot defied death that day, but not everyone is so lucky.

THE NO. 1 KILLER

What is the No. 1 killer of both men and women in the United States? It isn't cancer. It isn't traffic accidents. It isn't gun violence. It's coronary heart disease (CHD). Every 43 seconds an American dies from a coronary event. That's more than 2,000 deaths per day. And every year an estimated 735,000 Americans suffer a heart attack, also known as a myocardial infarction (MI), according to the American Heart Association (AHA).

The devastating and debilitating effects of CHD reach far beyond U.S. borders. CHD claims more lives worldwide than any other cause, and it is responsible for about one-third of all deaths in people over the age of 35. A 2014 World Health Organization study of 49 countries found that CHD was the culprit in over 4 million deaths that year.

If you or a loved one is living with CHD, you're not alone. Roughly one-half of middle-aged men and one-third of middle-aged women have some form of CHD. According to a long-term research project known as the Framingham Heart Study, which followed more than 5,200 people between age 30 and 62 for over 40 years, the incidence of coronary events is generally higher in men than in women. After women complete menopause, however, the incidence of CHD tends to even out between the sexes.

Although coronary events are more common in older Americans, this insidious disease can take root in the body many years or even decades before old age. According to the most recent AHA estimates, 16.5 million people over age 20 currently show signs of the disease.

If your doctor has diagnosed you with coronary heart disease or if you've suffered a heart attack, you likely have a lot of questions: Why did this happen to me? What treatments are available? What can I do to prevent a heart attack?

One of the first things you should do to protect yourself from a coronary event is to learn as much as you can about the disease, its causes, risk factors, treatment options, and recommended lifestyle changes. With knowledge on your side, you and your doctor can make the best decisions for your heart health.

YOUR AMAZING HEART

Your heart is an amazing pump that beats more than 100,000 times a day, every day of your life. That adds up to about 2.5 billion beats in a lifetime. Although it weighs less than a pound and is only about the size of a fist, your heart handles one of your body's most important processes: circulating blood throughout your body. Each minute, your heart pumps 1.5 gallons of blood, which adds up to over 2,000 gallons per day.

Located slightly left of center in the chest behind the breastbone, the heart has four chambers—two upper ones (the atriums or atria) and two lower ones (the ventricles). Divided in half by a thin membrane called the septum, the heart's chambers work in concert to keep blood flowing in the following endless sequence:

- The left atrium receives oxygenated blood from the lungs and pumps it to the left ventricle.
- The left ventricle pumps oxygen-rich blood to the organs in the body.
- The right atrium receives deoxygenated blood from the veins and pumps it to the right ventricle.
- The right ventricle receives blood from the right atrium and pumps it to the lungs, where it is oxygenated.

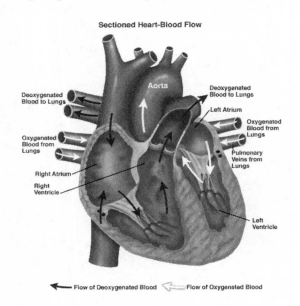

Sectioned Heart-Blood Flow

Deoxygenated Blood to Lungs

Aorta

Deoxygenated Blood to Lungs

Left Atrium

Oxygenated Blood from Lungs

Oxygenated Blood from Lungs

Pulmonary Veins from Lungs

Right Atrium

Right Ventricle

Left Ventricle

Flow of Deoxygenated Blood   Flow of Oxygenated Blood

The human heart can perform this continuous pumping action because it is a muscle, although it isn't like the other muscles in your body. Composed of smooth tissue, the heart pumps involuntarily, meaning you never have to think about it. The other approximately 700 skeletal muscles in your body are composed of voluntary tissue, which means they are controlled consciously. For example, you have to consciously think about walking to engage your quadriceps, hamstrings, and other leg muscles. You have to make a conscious decision to raise a glass of water to your mouth to spark the contraction of your biceps. You have to will yourself to do a sit-up to fire up your abdominal muscles. But you don't have to tell your heart to pump. It just keeps on beating.

The heart muscle also differs from skeletal muscles regarding healing and repair. Let's say you're playing in your company softball game, and it's your turn at bat. The pitcher tosses a juicy strike to you and you swing with everything you've got, hitting a blistering line drive past the third baseman. You drop the bat and start running toward first base when—*ouch!*—you pull your hamstring. You have to sit on the bench the rest of the game with an ice bag on the back of your thigh. Almost immediately, inside your body, your cells shift into repair mode to begin the healing process on that hamstring. With rest and time, your hamstring will be as good as new and you'll be back on the playing field.

Unfortunately, if you were playing in that same softball game and suffered a heart attack after you hit the ball, your cells wouldn't rush into repair mode. The heart simply does not heal or regenerate tissue the way skeletal muscles do. This is why it is so important to try to avoid damage to the heart muscle.

THE CIRCULATORY SYSTEM

The heart is just one part of the body's circulatory system, also known as the cardiovascular system. This system includes the lungs as well as blood vessels called arteries, veins, and capillaries. Arteries transport blood, oxygen, and nourishment from the heart to the body, and veins carry deoxygenated blood back to the heart. Tiny blood vessels called capillaries form connections between arteries and veins.

Circulatory System

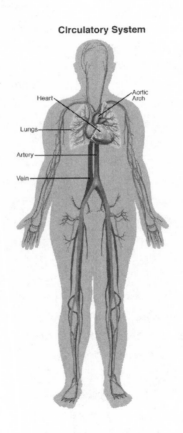

The circulatory system is vast. In fact, if you laid all the blood vessels in your body end to end, they would measure approximately 60,000 miles, more than twice the circumference of the earth or about 10 round trips from Los Angeles to New York City.

The circulatory system is similar to the nation's highway system. Think of the blood vessels in your body as a complex network of one-way highways and roads. Oxygen-rich blood, which is bright red in color, travels through the arteries to the body's organs. After nourishing the organs, the oxygen-depleted blood, now dark red, picks up waste and debris and returns to the heart via the veins. In between, capillaries act like bridges shuttling blood between the arteries and veins.

Your circulatory system can move blood through your body surprisingly quickly. Just like with real highways, the wider the artery, the faster traffic flows; the smaller the throughway, the slower it goes. On average, blood flows at about 3 to 4 miles per hour—average walking speed. If a nurse injects a drug into your arm, though, it can reach your brain in a matter of seconds.

All this internal circulation happens 24/7 every day of the year—whether you're playing softball, watching TV on the couch, or reading a book.

CORONARY ARTERIES

Just like all the other organs in your body, your heart relies on oxygenated blood to work properly. Its supply of nourishment comes from two main coronary arteries that rise from the base of the aorta, the largest artery in the human body.

The two vessels that branch off from the aorta to feed the heart are called the left main (LM) and the right coronary artery (RCA). The LM further divides into two branches, the left anterior descending (LAD) artery and the left circumflex (LCX) artery. The LAD artery supplies oxygenated blood to the front outer side of the septum, while the LCX artery carries blood to the back and bottom of the heart. The RCA, meanwhile, shuttles blood to the right atrium, right ventricle, and lower back part of the left ventricle.

The health of these arteries is critical to the heart's ability to perform its job. Healthy coronary arteries have smooth, flexible walls that allow blood to flow freely through them.

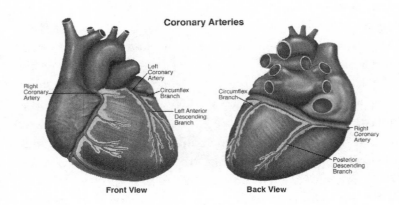

Coronary Arteries

Front View   Back View

WHAT LEADS TO CORONARY HEART DISEASE?

You may think coronary heart disease is a product of our modern lifestyle, but it has been found in 3,000-year-old mummies. In all the years since then, we have learned that a process called atherosclerosis leads to CHD, also known as coronary artery disease (CAD). This process causes the inner walls of the coronary arteries to become damaged, narrowed, and clogged.

The disease, which may begin as early as childhood in people who are predisposed to the condition, starts out as a little fatty streak on the innermost wall of the coronary artery. The fatty streak gets larger as cholesterol is deposited, eventually becoming a plaque inside the artery. As time goes by, the plaque begins to grow and calcify. This process is similar to the way minerals and other materials build up in the pipes in your home. As the buildup grows, the pipes become clogged, and the water no longer flows as freely as it should. The water may even stop running completely.

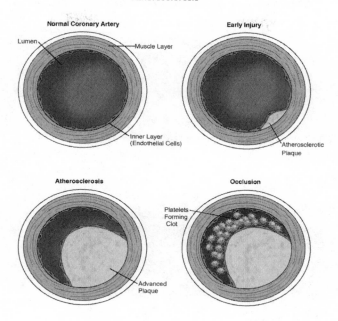

Atherosclerosis

A comparable process can happen in your arteries. The thickening plaque may cause arteries to narrow, reducing the amount of oxygenated blood that reaches your heart. This can lead to chest pain or pressure called angina. If the plaque buildup obstructs the artery completely, it will cut off the oxygen supply, which will result in a heart attack. As plaques grow, they become more calcified. People who have high levels of calcium in their arteries are believed to be at higher risk of a coronary event.

In some cases, a plaque may grow and rupture. The dislodged plaque stimulates the formation of a blood clot, a clump of blood that has transformed from liquid form to a more gel-like consistency. This can lead to chest pain, heart attack, or even death.

Other factors play a critical role in the formation of a clot. If the artery's inner wall, called the endothelium, becomes injured or diseased, it sends an SOS signal throughout the blood vessel. Then the blood vessel's emergency repair squad, composed of platelets, goes into action. These tiny particles, which have an average lifespan of only seven to 10 days, rush to the damaged area and start clumping together in an attempt to patch it. In some people, however, the platelets continue clumping even after completing the repair. This excessive repair work leads to the formation of a platelet-rich clot, or thrombus.

Clot Formation

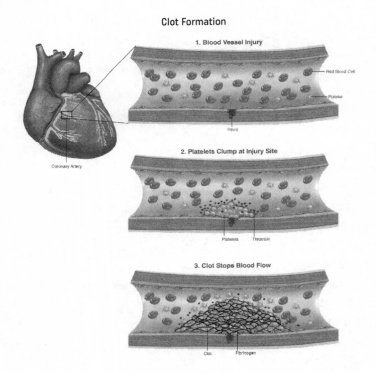

Another cause of CAD involves a different substance present in blood called thrombin. Thrombin senses when there is damage to the inner wall of an artery and recruits and activates platelets as well as a protein in the blood called fibrinogen. Like platelets, fibrinogen contributes to blood clotting, which can block an artery. Partial blockage of an artery can lead to chest pain, whereas a complete blockage will result in a heart attack, which can damage the muscle. In some cases, the extent of the damage is so great that the heart can no longer perform, leading to death. In many cases, however, the harm is minor or moderate and can be managed.

ACUTE CORONARY SYNDROME AND HEART ATTACK

Every year, approximately 120,000 people die from a heart attack—but more than 600,000 survive. In part, that's because not all heart attacks are the same. Healthcare professionals use an umbrella term, "acute coronary syndrome" (ACS), to describe cardiac events that constitute medical emergencies. Your chances of surviving ACS depend on many factors, including the type of cardiac event you experience. ACS includes:

Unstable angina: Unstable angina is the acute onset of severe chest pain or prolonged chest pain not associated with physical exertion. This condition puts you at greater risk of heart attack.

STEMI: An ST-segment elevation myocardial infarction (STEMI) is a type of heart attack that involves a complete blockage in at least one artery. It is associated with specific EKG changes easily recognized by healthcare professionals. STEMI puts the heart muscle at major risk of damage.

NSTEMI: A non-ST-segment elevation myocardial infarction (NSTEMI) is a heart attack involving one or more partial blockages in the arteries. It is not associated with easily recognizable EKG changes. Depending on the severity of the partial blockages, it may cause damage to the heart muscle.

Sudden cardiac arrest: This catastrophic condition, often due to a sudden heart attack, occurs when the heart unexpectedly stops beating, causing a person to pass out and stop breathing. Almost 70 percent of deaths from heart disease result from sudden cardiac arrest.

WHAT CAUSES ATHEROSCLEROSIS?

Atherosclerosis is the most studied disease in the Western world, yet its direct causes remain elusive. What medical experts have been able to glean from thousands of research studies is that this process often begins early in life and progresses with age. Within the medical community, it is believed that the following conditions may contribute to atherosclerosis:

- Elevated levels of low-density lipoprotein (LDL) cholesterol
- Low levels of high-density lipoprotein (HDL) cholesterol
- Elevated levels of lipoprotein(a), a particle in the blood that carries cholesterol
- Elevated levels of homocysteine
- Elevated levels of triglycerides
- High blood pressure
- Smoking
- Family history of premature CAD (under age 55 in men and 65 in women)
- Diabetes mellitus
- Obesity
- Chronic inflammation

Medical experts believe that the process of atherosclerosis likely involves a combination of these conditions. Some of these factors are genetic, but having a predisposition for CAD does not mean you will definitely develop the disease. Although some risk factors, such as your age and genetics, are nonmodifiable, many others are modifiable. Diabetes, high blood pressure, smoking, obesity, and an unhealthy lifestyle, for example, are all within your power to change and control.

CHAPTER 2

KNOW YOUR RISK LEVEL

I have a friend—an internist at one of the hospitals where I work—who is the epitome of physical health. At 45, Martin is very lean and plays high-level racquetball, runs, watches his diet, and has never smoked. One morning, he got up at his usual early hour, threw on his running gear, and went out for a quick jog in a local park. He came back home, did a few stretches, and ate some breakfast. Then he started feeling like he had indigestion. That wasn't unusual for him, so he popped a couple antacids. After a few hours, the indigestion hadn't gone away. Martin thought he might be having an issue with his gallbladder, so he drove himself to the ER at the hospital where he works and asked a colleague to run a few tests to check his gallbladder.

The tests showed that Martin's gallbladder was fine. That was the good news. The bad news was that his EKG was highly abnormal, indicating ACS. More specifically, it meant Martin was having a heart attack. That's when he was whisked into the cath lab. I performed a heart catheterization on him and discovered that Martin had several blockages in his arteries. I called in the cardiovascular surgeon, and the next day we performed a quadruple bypass on him. That was 15 years ago. Today, Martin is back to his usual picture of health and still plays racquetball and runs.

After his heart attack, Martin wanted my help to figure out why it had happened. He thought he was doing everything right to protect his health, and he had no history of any heart problems, so he couldn't understand why he fell victim to a heart attack. We went through a list of risk factors—high blood pressure, diabetes, and more—and he didn't have any of them. Then I asked him about his family history. That's when he told me his brother had been diagnosed with coronary heart disease at age 39. I informed him that having a first-degree family member with premature heart disease is a major risk factor for CHD. I told him that if I had known about his brother, I would have insisted that Martin come to see me sooner to have his heart health tested. If he had, he might have avoided that heart attack and the bypass surgery.

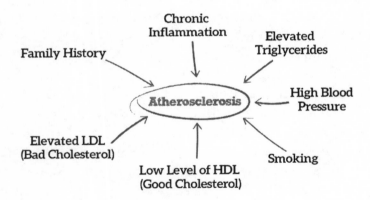

ARE YOU AT RISK?

If you've been told you have coronary heart disease or you've had a heart attack, you may wonder what put you at risk. Was it a genetic predisposition you inherited from your grandfather? Was it because you have high blood pressure? Was it because you have a very stressful job? Was it all that pizza you ate in college? The medical community has been searching for the answers to these questions for decades. Although we cannot predict with 100 percent certainty who will have a heart attack and who will not, we have identified certain conditions and lifestyle choices that can make a person more likely to develop CHD. These are called risk factors.

In general, having more risk factors increases the likelihood of developing CHD. Based on thousands of research studies and decades of data, the American Heart Association and the American College of Cardiology have identified the following as the strongest predictors for 10-year risk of developing CHD: older age, male gender, race, elevated total cholesterol, low HDL "good" cholesterol, high blood pressure, blood pressure treatment status, diabetes, and smoking. When assessing the risk of CHD, cardiologists also take into account a number of other factors.

Top Risk Factors for CHD and Heart Attack

- Older age
- Male gender
- Race and ethnicity
- Elevated levels of total cholesterol
- Low levels of good cholesterol
- High blood pressure
- Blood pressure treatment status
- Diabetes
- Smoking

Being aware of these factors and knowing your personal risk level is an important step in understanding the disease. Controlling your risk factors may slow the growth of atherosclerotic plaques, reverse disease, or even prevent a heart attack.

OLDER AGE

Most of us associate getting older with the appearance of a sprinkling of gray hairs, a few more lines on our faces, and an invitation to join

AARP. But there's another thing that comes with age: an increased risk of heart disease. Although CHD and heart attack can strike at any age, your risk rises as you get older. In men, the risk begins to increase after reaching age 45. From age 35 to 44, some 25 men per 1,000 suffer a heart attack or die from CHD. That number jumps to 75 per 1,000 in men between the ages of 45 and 54 and continues to skyrocket from age 55 to 74, when the rate reaches 125 men per 1,000.

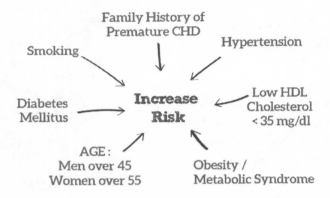

Coronary Heart Disease (CHD) Risk Factors

Family History of Premature CHD

Smoking

Hypertension

Diabetes Mellitus → **Increase Risk** ← Low HDL Cholesterol < 35 mg/dl

AGE: Men over 45 Women over 55

Obesity / Metabolic Syndrome

In women, the risk goes up once they hit age 55 and especially after menopause. Only 35 women per 1,000 suffer a heart attack or fatal CHD from age 45 to 54. Starting at age 55, however, that number hits 60 per 1,000, and it continues to rise for the rest of a woman's life, eventually outpacing men after age 85.

MALE GENDER

Being male increases your risk of having CHD or a coronary event such as a heart attack. This elevated risk continues until age 85, when a man's risk falls below a woman's risk. It is unclear what causes the increased risk in the male gender. Most likely, the presence of estrogen in women offers some protection against CHD. Current data show that women's risk levels become the same as men's after menopause, or about age 55, when their estrogen levels drop.

RACE AND ETHNICITY

Race and ethnicity may play a role in your risk of coronary heart disease, heart attack, and death from CHD. For example, death rates from CHD are 33 percent higher among African-Americans than the general population. Native Americans and Alaska Natives are more likely to die from CHD at a younger age than other ethnicities, with 36 percent dying before reaching age 65 compared with 17 percent of the overall U.S. population. Asians who have low levels of HDL "good" cholesterol experience a higher level of coronary events compared with the general population.

Many believe the reasons some racial groups and ethnicities experience higher rates of CHD and heart attack relate to higher incidences of risk factors, such as diabetes, high blood pressure, and obesity. In addition, some ethnic minorities may confront greater barriers to quality medical care and early diagnosis. A lack of access to health insurance or quality care can result in more advanced disease and worse outcomes.

FAMILY HISTORY

Did your mother have a heart attack? Does your brother have CHD? If your parents or siblings have been diagnosed with CHD or experienced a heart attack, you are at an increased risk of developing the disease. This family predisposition for CHD is strongest among first-degree relatives—your parents and siblings—and not as pronounced with more distant relatives, such as cousins, aunts, and uncles. In particular, if your family members were diagnosed with premature heart disease—father or brother under 55 years of age, mother or sister under 65 years of age—your risk level rises.

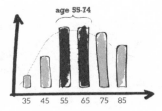

Men

Men are more likely to suffer from coronary heart disease (CHD) earlier in life than women.

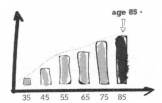

Women

Women's risk of CHD gets progressively higher after age 55 and surpasses men's risk after age 85.

In my own practice, I have noticed that family history tends to affect males more than females. So if a father was diagnosed with premature CHD, his sons appear to be more likely to be affected than his daughters. In such families, women do not tend to develop CHD. However, in some families both sexes are afflicted.

If you have a family history of heart disease, you may have inherited genes that make you more prone to some of the underlying risk factors for the disease, such as high blood pressure, diabetes, or high cholesterol. Your family environment may also affect your risk level. Being raised by parents who smoke, for example, can increase your chances of becoming a smoker. Growing up in a house full of overeaters can have a detrimental effect on your own lifelong eating habits. When you combine genetic factors with unhealthy lifestyle habits, you compound your risk.

UNHEALTHY CHOLESTEROL LEVELS

If you watch TV news or glance at health and nutrition magazines at the grocery store, you're probably aware that cholesterol often makes headlines. You may know that egg yolks are high in dietary cholesterol or that many people take prescription medicine called statins to lower their cholesterol. Your doctor may even have advised you to lower your cholesterol. That's because having high cholesterol levels is one of the major underlying causes of CHD.

According to the decades-long Framingham Heart Study, elevated levels of cholesterol increase the risk of CHD. Yet cholesterol is not inherently bad for you. In fact, cholesterol, a waxy substance that exists in every cell in your body, performs many important functions, such as helping produce hormones and vitamins and helping you digest foods.

Where does cholesterol come from? Your body gets it from two sources: your liver and the foods you eat. Your liver naturally produces the cholesterol your body needs to perform these important functions. Consuming certain types of foods that contain saturated fats and trans fats—foods made with partially hydrogenated vegetable oils—can cause your liver to produce additional cholesterol. In particular, foods like thick steaks, gooey cheese, and store-bought cookies are associated with increased production of cholesterol, which can lead to elevated levels that put you at higher risk of CHD.

The cholesterol in your body needs to travel through your bloodstream to perform its primary duties, but it cannot do so on its own. Fatty, waxy cholesterol does not dissolve in your blood; it needs to hitch a ride to make it through your circulatory system. Complexes called lipoproteins, which act like cargo carriers, surround the cholesterol and take it on its voyage through your blood vessels.

Cardiologists have identified several types of cholesterol: LDL (low-density lipoprotein), HDL (high-density lipoprotein), VLDL (very low-density lipoprotein), chylomicrons, and LP(a) (lipoprotein a).

LDL: This lipoprotein is considered "bad" cholesterol. Think of the "L" in LDL as "lousy." LDL is like a litterbug who throws a lot of trash along the highway as it drives. LDL travels through your bloodstream, leaving deposits of fatty cholesterol that contribute to the buildup of plaque in the arteries. The more LDL you have circulating in your blood, the more trash that gets deposited in your arteries. As you have seen, plaque formation can lead to CHD and heart attack, so having high levels of LDL raises your risk.

HDL: This is the so-called "good" cholesterol. Think of the "H" in HDL as "happy." HDL is like your personal trash collector. It travels through your bloodstream, picking up the excess cholesterol that has been deposited on the artery walls and carrying it back to your liver for elimination. In this way, HDL helps prevent, slow, or even reverse the formation of plaque. The more HDL you have in your blood, the lower your risk of disease.

VLDL: This lipoprotein transports cholesterol as well as another type of fat known as triglycerides. Medical experts believe that high levels of triglycerides may contribute to plaque formation and increase your risk of CHD and heart attack.

Chylomicrons: After eating a fatty meal—think cheeseburgers, pizza, or ice cream—your liver produces this type of lipoprotein to transport the dietary cholesterol as well as triglycerides through your body.

LP(a): This type of lipoprotein transports cholesterol, fats, and protein in your blood vessels. The amount of LP(a) your body produces is inherited from your parents. Some people naturally produce high levels of this substance, which adds to your risk. Approximately 63 million Americans have high levels of LP(a), and these individuals have two to four times the risk of developing early CHD. LP(a) levels tend to remain constant throughout a person's lifetime and do not appear to be affected by diet or exercise.

Your overall risk of CHD depends on which type of cholesterol you have in your body. When assessing your risk, doctors primarily look at LDL, HDL, triglycerides, and LP(a). Having high levels of LDL, triglycerides, and LP(a) or low levels of the protective HDL increases your risk. Because cholesterol levels have been shown to play such an important role in your risk of CHD, it's important to know your numbers. If you're over the age of 20, you should have your cholesterol levels checked every four to six years, according to AHA recommendations. A complete lipoprotein profile will typically include your blood levels of total cholesterol, LDL, HDL, triglycerides, and LP(a).

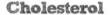

Cholesterol

TOTAL, LDL, & HDL Cholesterol:
Where should each of your
numbers be?

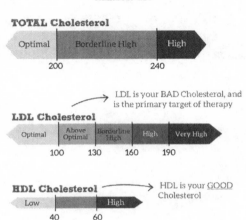

Total Cholesterol Levels

(Measurements are given in milligrams per deciliter. Note that for people with CHD or who have more than two risk factors, the desired levels may be lower. Speak to your doctor to determine your optimal levels.)

Less than 200	Optimal
200-239	Borderline high
240 or above	High

LDL "Bad" Cholesterol Levels

(Measurements are given in milligrams per deciliter. Note that for people with CHD or who have more than two risk factors, the desired levels may be lower. Speak to your doctor to determine your optimal levels.)

Less than 100	Optimal
100-129	Near optimal/above optimal
130-159	Borderline high
160-189	High
190 or above	Very high

HDL "Good" Cholesterol Levels

(Measurements are given in milligrams per deciliter. Note that for people with CHD or who have more than two risk factors, the desired levels may be higher. Speak to your doctor to determine your optimal levels.)

60 or above	Considered protective against CHD
40-59	Not a major risk factor for CHD
Less than 40	A major risk factor for CHD

Triglycerides Levels

(Measurements are given in milligrams per deciliter. Note that for people with CHD or who have more than two risk factors, the desired levels may be lower. Speak to your doctor to determine your optimal levels.)

Less than 150	Normal
150-199	Borderline high
200-499	High
500 or above	Very high

LP(a) Levels

(Measurements are given in milligrams per deciliter.)

Less than 30   Normal

30 or above   Higher risk

HIGH BLOOD PRESSURE

Blood pressure is a measurement of the pressure created within your arteries as blood pumps through them. Blood pressure is expressed in two numbers—systolic (top number) and diastolic (bottom number)—and is given in millimeters of mercury (mmHg). As you saw in Chapter 1, every time your heart beats—more than 100,000 times per day—it pushes blood into your arteries. The force of that blood hitting the inner walls of your arteries is your systolic blood pressure. The pressure in your vessels between heartbeats is your diastolic blood pressure.

When the force in your vessels is too high, it is called hypertension or high blood pressure. One of the most common chronic conditions in the U.S., hypertension affects approximately 50 million Americans. When you have high blood pressure, your heart must work harder. Because of this, hypertension can eventually cause thickening of the heart muscle. Studies show that having high blood pressure roughly doubles the risk of death due to a coronary event in both men and women. In fact, in adults ages 40 to 89, the risk of death from a coronary event doubles with every increase of 20 points systolic or 10 points diastolic blood pressure.

Surprisingly, high blood pressure produces no symptoms, which means you could have hypertension for years without realizing it. The only way to diagnose hypertension is to have your blood pressure taken by a medical professional. Because hypertension is a major risk factor for heart disease, it is critical that all adults have their blood pressure checked on a regular basis.

In 2017, the American College of Cardiology and the American Heart Association released new guidelines for the first time since 2003 that lower the definition of high blood pressure. The new guidelines allow for earlier intervention with lifestyle changes and, in some cases, medication. The ACC and AHA recognize five categories of blood pressure: normal, elevated, stage 1, stage 2, and hypertensive crisis.

Normal: If your blood pressure is in the normal range, continue following a heart-healthy diet and exercising on a regular basis.

Elevated: If your blood pressure is elevated, you are more likely to develop hypertension in the future. Taking steps to control it now can help prevent it from progressing.

Stage 1: At this stage, your doctor may recommend lifestyle changes, such as following the DASH diet (a low-sodium eating plan that emphasizes an increase in foods rich in potassium and calcium), reducing alcohol intake to no more than two drinks per day, and increasing physical activity. In some cases, medication may be prescribed to lower your blood pressure.

Stage 2: When hypertension reaches this stage, doctors typically prescribe blood pressure medicine in addition to lifestyle changes.

Hypertensive Crisis: If blood pressure reaches this level and does not go down within a few minutes, it can be an emergency situation. Call 911.

Blood Pressure Levels
(Numbers are expressed in millimeters of mercury, or mmHg.)

Category	Systolic (upper #)	Diastolic (lower #)
Normal	Less than 120	Less than 80
Elevated	120-129	Less than 80
Stage 1	130-139	80-89
Stage 2	140+	90+
Hypertensive Crisis	180+	120+

DIABETES

Diabetes mellitus is a condition in which the body can't adequately produce or respond to the hormone insulin, resulting in elevated blood glucose levels. Produced in the pancreas, insulin helps your body transfer sugar in the bloodstream to your cells, where it is used for energy. When your body doesn't produce enough insulin or doesn't respond properly to the insulin—a condition known as insulin resistance—the sugar remains in your bloodstream rather than being converted into energy.

Approximately 21 million people in the U.S. have been diagnosed with diabetes, while millions more are likely living with the disease but don't know it. Diabetes is rapidly becoming more prevalent in the U.S. and around the world. In 1985, an estimated 30 million people worldwide had the disease. Experts project that by 2025 that number will explode to 350 million.

These numbers include two types of diabetes: Type 1 and Type 2. Type 1 diabetes, often diagnosed in young children and once known as juvenile diabetes, means the pancreas simply does not produce insulin. People diagnosed with Type 1 diabetes typically require insulin injections for the remainder of their lifetime. Type 2 diabetes, which is more common and usually develops later in life, can indicate either a lack of insulin production or the body's inability to respond to the hormone.

Both Type 1 and Type 2 diabetes put you at greater risk of CHD and heart attack. In fact, approximately 70 to 80 percent of all people with CHD have been diagnosed with diabetes or abnormal glucose tolerance. In addition, people with diabetes are two to eight times more likely to develop CHD than people without the condition. Diabetes accelerates the natural progression of atherosclerosis, which is why it is considered one of the strongest risk factors for CHD and heart attack.

As a general rule, people with Type 1 diabetes tend to have worse outcomes following coronary events than those with Type 2 diabetes. Women with either type have almost twice the risk of dying from a coronary event than men with diabetes.

How do you know if you have diabetes? The disease can be diagnosed with blood tests, such as a fasting glucose test or an A1c test, or with an oral glucose tolerance test.

Fasting glucose test: This reports the level of glucose in your blood at the time your blood is drawn. Higher numbers indicate a problem.

A1c test: This test provides an average of blood glucose levels over three months. It is often used to diagnose prediabetes and Type 2 diabetes, and provides information on how well a person is managing the disease.

Oral glucose tolerance test: For this test you fast overnight, then have your blood drawn to measure your glucose levels. Afterwards you drink a sugary beverage, then have your glucose levels tested a number of times in the following two hours. High levels of glucose in your blood after two hours indicate that your body has a problem converting sugar to energy.

Fasting Glucose Blood Test

(Measurements are expressed as milligrams per deciliter.)

Less than 100	Normal
100–125	Prediabetes
126 or above	Diabetes

A1c Blood Glucose Levels

(Measurements are expressed as percentages.)

5.7 or below	Normal
5.7–6.4	Prediabetes
6.5 or above	Diabetes

Oral Glucose Tolerance Test
(Measurements are expressed as milligrams per deciliter.)

Less than 140   Normal
140-199   Prediabetes
200 or above   Diabetes

Because diabetes is such a strong risk factor for CHD, it is very important to get regular screenings of your blood glucose levels. If you have diabetes, it is absolutely critical to control it with diet, exercise, and medication if prescribed.

OBESITY

Look at any magazine at the checkout stand in the grocery store and you'll see headlines like: "5 Tricks to Get Thinner," "10 Super-Slimming Foods for Summer," or "Get 6-Pack Abs in 6 Minutes a Day." Visit a bookstore and you'll find shelves full of diet books promising to give you the secrets to losing weight and keeping it off. Americans are obsessed with losing weight and spend billions each year trying to shed excess pounds. Despite all our efforts, we're gaining weight. Approximately two-thirds of Americans—that's more than 100 million people—are overweight or obese. From 1980 to 2013, the percentage of men worldwide who are obese has risen from 28.8 percent to 36.9 percent. Even more women have become obese, going from 29.8 percent in 1980 to 38 percent in 2013.

This is bad news for the heart. Obesity, recognized as a chronic disease by the American Medical Association, is associated with increased risks of developing CHD. This is partly due to the fact that being obese is also associated with a higher prevalence of glucose intolerance, insulin resistance, high blood pressure, physical inactivity, and high cholesterol—all factors that put you at greater risk of CHD.

31

Obesity is determined by your Body Mass Index (BMI), which is calculated by dividing your weight in kilograms by your height in meters. Having a BMI over 30 is considered obese. People who are morbidly obese, indicated by a BMI of 40 or higher, are at a much greater risk of having a heart attack and at a much younger age than average.

In addition to your BMI, your waist-to-hip ratio can also play a role in your risk of CHD. People who are thicker through the midsection tend to have higher death rates from heart disease compared with those who carry more weight around the hips and thighs. To calculate your waist-to-hip ratio, divide the circumference of your waist (measured at the smallest part of your waist) by the circumference of your hips (measured at the largest part of your hips). A waist-to-hip ratio of 0.8 or below for women and 0.95 or below for men is considered optimal.

Body Mass Index (BMI) Categories

Underweight: less than 18.5
Normal weight: 18.5-24.9
Overweight: 25-29.9
Obese: 30 or higher
Morbidly obese: 40 or higher

Waist-to-Hip Categories

Health Risk	Women	Men
Low	0.8 or below	0.95 or below
Moderate	0.81-0.85	0.96-1.0
High	0.86 or above	1.0 or above

In my practice, I see many patients who fall into the obese category on the BMI chart. But there is one man who really stands out in my mind. When Gary showed up in my office, he was 51 and at 5'10," he weighed more than 400 pounds. That put his BMI at over 57, more than double the normal BMI of less than 25. Gary was a mess. He was taking multiple prescription medications for high blood pressure, diabetes, and high cholesterol, and he occasionally had chest pains. I did a series of diagnostic tests and discovered that Gary had narrowing in one of his arteries, so I put a stent in to help alleviate his chest pain.

The whole experience hit Gary hard. He didn't want to die. He decided to get serious and began making small changes to his eating habits. He also started walking—just a few blocks at first, which grew into several miles a day. Less than two years later, Gary came back to see me for a follow-up visit. I didn't recognize him. He had lost over 200 pounds. I couldn't have been more proud of him. He looked like a new man—energetic and happy.

At 170 pounds now, his BMI was just under 25, which put him in the normal range. His diabetes was under control, and his cholesterol was in the healthy range, so he no longer needed medication for those conditions. He was down to taking one medication for his blood pressure. The real test would come when he got on the treadmill for a stress EKG. Gary hit the treadmill, and as he walked briskly on an uphill grade, his EKG looked perfectly healthy—no signs of heart disease.

In the 10 years since his first visit with me, Gary has passed his stress tests with flying colors. I love telling my other patients about Gary because he is a great example to show that with some effort, you can reverse CHD and improve your heart health.

METABOLIC SYNDROME

Metabolic syndrome is a cluster of medical conditions that boosts your chances of developing CHD and increases the likelihood of dying from it. In the U.S., an estimated 37 percent of the population has metabolic syndrome. The prevalence is even higher in other parts of the world; for example, 46 percent of the population in India has the condition.

To be diagnosed with metabolic syndrome, you must have at least three of the following conditions: abdominal obesity, high triglycerides, low levels of HDL cholesterol, high blood pressure, and high fasting blood sugar levels. As you have seen, each of these conditions on their own can contribute to CHD, but when a person has the cluster of conditions known as metabolic syndrome, it increases the risk even more.

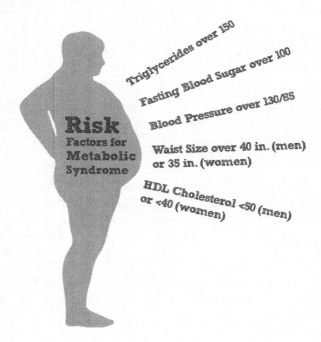

Risk
Factors for
Metabolic
Syndrome

Triglycerides over 150

Fasting Blood Sugar over 100

Blood Pressure over 130/85

Waist Size over 40 in. (men) or 35 in. (women)

HDL Cholesterol <50 (men) or <40 (women)

CHRONIC INFLAMMATORY DISEASE

Have you ever gotten a splinter in your finger? After you pull it out, the surrounding skin turns red and the area gets inflamed. After a few days, the swelling goes down and your skin returns to normal. This is your immune system's natural reaction to defend itself against foreign objects like splinters. Your immune system also kicks into action to fight viruses and bacteria.

In some people, conditions like high blood pressure or the presence of too much LDL cholesterol may cause damage in the blood vessels or heart that triggers the immune system to react, leading to inflammation. Sometimes the immune system gets stuck in fighting mode and inflammation becomes chronic.

Medical experts are still investigating how chronic inflammation affects the heart, but they have noted an association between the condition and CHD. Doctors have identified two indicators of high inflammation levels: high homocysteine levels and elevated C-reactive protein (CRP) levels.

High homocysteine levels: Homocysteine is an amino acid found in your blood. High levels of this substance are tied to a risk of developing CHD at an earlier age and are linked to low levels of certain B vitamins. Studies have shown that taking B vitamins can lower homocysteine levels, but that this has not resulted in a reduced risk of CHD.

Elevated CRP levels: Produced in the liver, CRP indicates inflammation in your body when its levels rise. Treating CRP with prescription medication can reduce the incidence of coronary events.

Homocysteine Levels

(Measurements are expressed as micromoles per liter.)

Normal	4-15
Moderate	15-30
Intermediate	30-100
Severe	100 and above

C-Reactive Protein (CRP) Levels
(Measurements are expressed as milligrams per liter.)

Low risk	less than 1.0
Intermediate risk	1.0-2.9
High risk	3.0 and above

CIGARETTE SMOKING

Everybody knows that cigarette smoking is associated with a higher incidence of lung cancer, but many people are unaware that it is also linked to a higher risk of heart disease, heart attack, and death from a coronary event. In the medical community, we have known about this link since 1964, when the Surgeon General's report first showed the adverse relationship between smoking and heart health. Since then, smoking has claimed 20 million lives in the U.S., and half a million Americans lose their lives every year to addictive cigarettes. Worldwide, 5 million to 6 million deaths annually are attributable to smoking.

In the mid-1960s, about 40 percent of the population smoked. By 2012, that number had dropped to about 12 percent. Even though the number of smokers is going down, about 1 billion people globally continue to light up. An estimated 800 million of them are men. People who smoke more than 20 cigarettes a day have a two- to threefold chance of developing CHD or having a heart attack.

We now understand the relationship between smoking and heart disease more clearly. Smoking decreases levels of HDL cholesterol, increases blood pressure, and makes blood more likely to form clots. In addition, cigarette smoke includes a mix of some 5,000 chemicals, many of which contain free radicals—compounds that damage cells and lead to inflammation. Nicotine, the addictive substance in cigarettes, is believed to be a major culprit in the development of atherosclerosis.

Even if you don't smoke, you may be vulnerable to increased risk if you have been exposed to secondhand smoke during your lifetime. For example, growing up with parents who smoked, having a roommate in college who smoked, or living with a spouse who smokes can put you at risk.

Smoking appears to have a more detrimental effect on the heart health of women than men. In particular, women who start smoking early in life experience a much higher incidence of heart disease at a younger age. Women smokers are also more likely to have blockages in the leg and neck arteries, which can lead to stroke. What's especially troubling is that although the overall number of smokers is declining, the number of female smokers in America is growing.

SEDENTARY LIFESTYLE

If you're the type of person who shuns physical activity and instead prefers to play video games, watch TV, or endlessly scroll through your social media accounts on your computer, then you're increasing your risk of CHD. Leading a sedentary lifestyle can make you more prone to becoming overweight and developing high blood pressure, inflammation, and diabetes.

MENTAL STRESS AND DEPRESSION

Many people are surprised to learn that physical conditions aren't the only risk factors associated with CHD. Having psychological conditions, such as depression or high levels of stress, can also contribute to the disease. About 1 in 10 American adults have depression, but approximately 1 in 3 heart attack patients also have a mental health condition. Some studies suggest that the correlation may be linked to the increased likelihood of engaging in unhealthy habits—eating junk food or skipping workouts, for example—when you are depressed. Similarly, experiencing excessive stress in your life may also lead to everyday behaviors that increase your risk.

ADDITIONAL RISK FACTORS

A number of other conditions and lifestyle habits contribute to CHD, although they are not considered strong risk factors. These contributing factors include:

- End-stage renal disease
- Low levels of testosterone
- Lack of sleep (less than five to six hours per night)
- Too much sleep (more than eight to nine hours per night)
- Cerebral vascular disease
- Peripheral arterial disease

MYTHBUSTER: CONDITIONS NOT ASSOCIATED WITH INCREASED RISK OF CHD

Eating eggs will give you a heart attack! Birth control pills will give you a heart attack! Drinking milk will give you a heart attack! At some point in your life, you have probably heard these dire warnings or read them on the internet. But these common refrains are untrue. They are myths that have been disproven by the medical community. In fact, research shows that many things people think cause heart disease actually do not contribute to it. Here are some of the most common myths people believe are risk factors of CHD:

- Oral contraceptives
- Chronic H. pylori
- Coffee consumption
- Milk or dairy products
- Foods fried with olive oil or sunflower oil
- Egg consumption (up to one per day is OK)
- High levels of potassium
- Low levels of magnesium

- HIV-positive status
- Mercury exposure

Knowing the real risk factors of CHD and controlling modifiable risks are two of the best ways to slow or reverse atherosclerosis and prevent a heart attack.

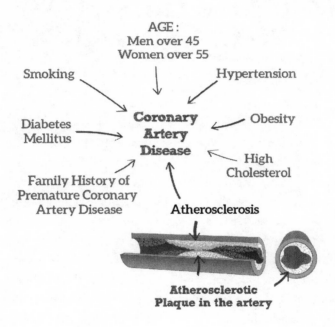

CHAPTER 3

RECOGNIZE THE SYMPTOMS AND WARNING SIGNS

If you're like most people, you probably think that having a heart attack is just like it's depicted in the movies: Someone dramatically clutches their chest in agony, then keels over. You might assume that crushing chest pain will make it obvious you're having a heart attack. Even though this happens in some instances, it isn't always the case. CHD and acute coronary syndrome (ACS), including heart attacks, can cause other, more subtle symptoms that you might not expect. That's what happened to Maureen.

A Texan in her mid-60s, Maureen and her husband planned to take their grandchildren out to dinner to celebrate their grandson's first win as quarterback of his high school football team. Before the big celebration, Maureen went about her typical day, tending to her expansive ranch and lifting heavy bales of hay to feed the horses. After a lifetime on the ranch, she was still very strong and fit for her age. That night, she and her husband, Bill, took the grandchildren to a steakhouse. Maureen didn't usually indulge in steak, but it was a special night, so she ordered a T-bone.

After dinner, her stomach hurt, and she started feeling queasy. She took some antacids, but they didn't help. The pain and nausea didn't go away. Then she started sweating profusely. Bill told her she should go to the hospital, but Maureen didn't want to make a big fuss about it. She was certain it was just the steak she ate. Bill insisted and brought her in. I was working in the hospital that night when Maureen arrived. Because we suspected ACS, we immediately did an EKG, which clearly showed that Maureen was having a heart attack. We started her on aspirin and took her to the cath lab for additional testing. There we discovered a big blockage in one of her arteries, so we put in a stent to get the blood flowing again.

Maureen was lucky we were able to open up her artery with a stent, but she was angry with herself for not going to the hospital sooner. She had convinced herself that her symptoms were due to the steak she had eaten. She isn't alone. Many people blame their symptoms on the chili, Mexican food, Chinese food, or other spicy food they ate that day. But in some cases, it isn't the food. It's a heart attack. Take the time to become familiar with the symptoms and warning signs of coronary heart disease and heart attack. It could save your life.

SYMPTOMS OF CHD, ACS, AND HEART ATTACK

Symptoms are clues your body gives you that something is wrong. CHD can produce a number of symptoms, but because the disease may develop slowly over time, it can be years before symptoms appear. As the disease progresses, arteries may narrow or blockages may appear that prevent adequate amounts of blood or oxygen from getting to your heart. A lack of sufficient oxygen to the heart can cause you to experience a variety of symptoms. In some cases, you may not have any symptoms until an artery is 70 to 80 percent blocked, but then the disease may progress rapidly, leading to a heart attack or death.

Chest Pain (Angina Pectoris)

By far, the most common symptom of CHD, ACS, and heart attack is chest pain, which cardiologists call angina pectoris or just angina. You may have a sensation of tightness, pressure, heaviness, burning, or pain in your chest. Some of my patients who are heart attack survivors say it feels like an elephant sitting on their chest. With angina, you can't make the pain worse by pressing your hand on the area, the way a bruise or pulled muscle would feel tender to the touch.

This type of chest pain is often triggered in situations when the heart muscle requires more oxygen, such as when you exert yourself. Exercise, cold weather, mental stress, and sexual activity all place heavier oxygen requirements on your heart. Angina has some unique characteristics:

- It is usually spread across the chest area rather than localized to one spot.
- It typically doesn't last for hours.
- It can last for just two to five minutes at a time.
- It may recur frequently.

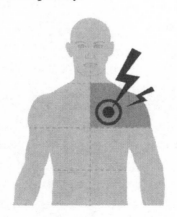

Chest Pain

Angina may be categorized as stable or unstable. Stable angina is predictable and often occurs with overexertion. You may feel it when you run uphill or when you do manual labor. Over time, you may become familiar with the activities or exertion levels that trigger angina.

If you have stable angina, but your chest pain becomes more severe, lasts longer than usual, or is triggered at lower levels of exertion—or if you have accompanying pain in other parts of the body or feel short of breath or dizzy—it is a sign that stable angina is becoming unstable angina. In this instance, seek medical attention immediately.

Unstable angina is not predictable. It may come on suddenly even when you aren't overexerting yourself and may be present when you are lying down or sleeping. This type of chest pain is considered ACS and requires emergency medical attention.

Radiating Pain and Referred Pain

Angina that is associated with CHD, ACS, and heart attack may also cause pain in other areas of the body. Some people experience discomfort in the jaw, neck, shoulders, arms, or back. This pain may accompany chest pain or may be present in the absence of angina. When you experience pain in the chest as well as other parts of the body, it is called radiating pain. If you feel pain in other areas, such as your jaw, back, or arm, but don't have any pain in your chest, it is called referred pain. This can occur when angina is referred to a nerve supply in the cervical spinal column that is connected to pain impulses.

WARNING SIGNS OF A HEART ATTACK

The most common warning sign of a heart attack is chest discomfort that may feel like pain, pressure, squeezing, tightness, or fullness. The pain may be sudden or may grow more slowly and

Common Warning Signs of a Heart Attack

- Chest discomfort, pain, or tightness
- Discomfort in jaw
- Discomfort in neck
- Discomfort in back
- Discomfort in arms
- Discomfort in stomach
- Shortness of breath
- Cold sweat
- Nausea
- Lightheadedness
- Extreme fatigue
- Sense of doom

often lasts more than a few minutes. Warning signs also include discomfort in other areas of the body, including the jaw, neck, back, arms, or stomach. You may feel numbness or tingling in the left shoulder and arm. Shortness of breath is a common warning sign of a heart attack. Breaking out in a cold sweat, feeling nauseated, feeling lightheaded, or feeling extreme fatigue are other warning signs. Many people suffering a heart attack also have a feeling of doom as if they are going to die.

If you think you're having a heart attack, call 911 immediately!

Women and Heart Attack Warning Signs

Although women in the U.S. are more likely to die of CHD than any other cause, they are less likely to have classic heart attack symptoms. For medical professionals, this can present a challenge. Some women who are having a heart attack complain of an achy, heavy, or burning sensation in the chest rather than typical pain. Some may have pain in their shoulders or in between their shoulder blades. Sometimes they just feel unusually tired or sick to their stomach. Others complain about difficulty breathing.

In general, women wait much longer than men to go to the ER when experiencing the warning signs of a heart attack. This puts them at greater risk of poorer outcomes. In fact, women are twice as likely to die in the hospital as men due to heart attack. Women tend to have heart attacks later in life than men—about 10 years later on average—however, women who have a heart attack before age 45 have a worse prognosis than men.

Common Heart Attack Warning Signs in Women

- Heaviness in chest
- Burning sensation in chest
- Achy feeling in chest
- Pain in shoulders
- Pain between shoulder blades
- Extreme fatigue
- Nausea
- Difficulty breathing

Younger People and Heart Attack Warning Signs

In younger people, a heart attack may not produce any symptoms at all. In fact, a higher proportion of younger patients don't experience any chest pain during a heart attack. Young people who are diagnosed with CHD are more likely to have rapid progression to a heart attack if treatment is delayed. When young people come to the hospital with chest pain, we test for CHD and heart attack, but we also check for drug use. Certain drugs, such as cocaine, can narrow arteries and lead to chest pain or heart attack.

SILENT HEART ATTACK

Did you know that you can have a heart attack and not even know it? In fact, about 20 percent of all heart attacks produce no symptoms. When a shortage of blood and oxygen to the heart doesn't produce any symptoms, it's called silent ischemia. The word "ischemia" is derived from the Latin word for "stopping." Silent ischemia may cause damage to your heart even though you are unaware of it. This type of heart attack is more common than you might imagine and may go undiagnosed. People with diabetes, for example, are more likely to have an asymptomatic heart attack.

IF IT ISN'T A HEART ATTACK, WHAT IS IT?

Although chest pain is the most common symptom of heart attack, it doesn't always mean you're having a coronary. Chest pain can be due to many other things.

Musculoskeletal pain: One of the more common causes of chest pain not associated with CHD is an issue with the muscles or bones in the chest wall. Trauma to the chest wall is often to blame. For example, if you were playing softball and the batter hit a line drive straight into your chest, it might hurt for a few days. If you got into a car accident, the force from the seatbelt preventing you from flying through the windshield might cause minor injuries to your internal chest muscles. Or, you may have cracked a rib when your doubles tennis partner accidentally whacked you in the side with their racquet. In general, this type of pain feels worse when you move—think bending over, twisting, or taking a deep breath. In addition, it tends to be localized, meaning you can pinpoint the painful area, and it hurts when you touch it or press on it.

Fibromyalgia: Feeling tenderness in the chest is a common symptom of fibromyalgia. However, this condition typically causes widespread musculoskeletal pain rather than discomfort in one area.

Rheumatoid arthritis: Chest discomfort is often experienced in people who have rheumatoid arthritis. This condition, associated with inflammation within the body, may cause diffuse pain throughout the body. It is uncommon for pain to be felt only in the chest.

Tietze's syndrome: This rare musculoskeletal disease causes pain in the ribcage and rib joints. It occurs due to swelling of the cartilage that connects the upper ribs to the breastbone.

Costochondritis: Another culprit of noncardiac chest pain is something called costochondritis. This pain emanates from the junctions where cartilage attaches to the ribs. With this condition, pressing on the area usually increases the pain.

Stomach problems: Pain in the chest or upper pit of stomach can be from gastrointestinal disease, a peptic ulcer, or gastroesophageal reflux disease (GERD). When this is the case, the pain can last up to an hour, intensifies when lying down, feels worse when you eat, and can be relieved with antacids. This type of pain does not radiate to the arm, neck, jaw, or back.

Esophageal spasm: In some cases, chest pain may arise because of a spasm in the esophagus. These spasms, which can last from five minutes to an hour, tend to be brought on when drinking cold liquids. Placing a nitroglycerin tablet under the tongue can help expand the esophagus to alleviate the pain.

Gallbladder disease: Pain on the lower right side of the chest may be caused by a diseased gallbladder. The gallbladder, a small pear-shaped organ that sits below the liver, plays a role in digestion. It stores bile, which is a substance that helps break down digestive fat in your small intestine. Pain is the most common symptom of a problem with the gallbladder. Eating food typically worsens the pain.

Lung problems: Chest pain that worsens when you take a deep breath, sneeze, or cough may be due to inflammation of the lungs' lining. A thin tissue-like membrane lines the lungs and the inner wall of the chest cavity. This protective lining is called the pleura, and when it becomes inflamed, it is referred to as pleurisy.

Pericarditis: Some chest pain is caused by inflammation of the heart lining. Your heart is surrounded by the pericardium, a sac-like structure consisting of two thin layers of tissue. When the pericardium becomes inflamed, its tissue can rub against the heart, causing pain that may be mistaken for a heart attack.

Collapsed lung: A collapsed lung, known as pneumothorax, can cause sudden chest pain and shortness of breath. When air leaks out of the lung into the chest cavity, the pressure of that air can cause the lung to collapse. Although this chest pain does not indicate a heart attack, it is a medical emergency and you should call 911 or go to the ER if you think you may be experiencing a collapsed lung.

Pulmonary embolism: A blood clot that travels to the lungs and blocks one of the arteries that feeds the lungs may cause sudden shortness of breath and chest pain. The pain typically worsens when you eat, breathe deeply, bend over, or cough. A blood clot in the lungs is a medical emergency that requires immediate attention.

Aortic dissection: A sudden stabbing pain in the chest may be due to a tear in the aorta, the main artery that carries blood from your heart to the rest of the organs in your body. When the aorta develops a hole, blood bursts out into the body with such force that it can split the layers of the artery wall, which is known as a dissection. Aortic dissection is a life-threatening emergency. If you suspect you are experiencing this condition, call 911.

Esophageal rupture: A tear in the esophagus can cause mild to severe chest pain. When there is a rupture in the esophagus, it allows food to leak out into the chest, which often causes lung problems. An esophageal rupture is a medical emergency. Seek treatment immediately.

Anxiety and panic attacks: Some people who have anxiety or who are experiencing a panic attack may fear that they are having a heart attack. They may have symptoms, such as tightness in the chest, lightheadedness, tingling sensations in the arms or legs, heart palpitations, dizziness, shortness of breath, or a feeling of doom. As you can see, these symptoms mirror many of those associated with a heart attack. If you are diagnosed with anxiety or panic attacks, work with your doctor or mental health professional to get your anxiety under control. With effective counseling and treatment, you may be able to recognize the onset of a panic attack and prevent it from progressing to the symptoms that mimic a heart attack.

STEPS TO SURVIVE A HEART ATTACK

Regardless of your age or gender, you can take certain measures to increase your chances of surviving a heart attack. First, remember

Common Causes for Non-Heart-Related Chest Pain

Condition	Time Duration of Symptoms
Gastroesophageal Reflux Disease (GERD) - worse laying down - exacerbated w/ food intake - no radiation - decreased w/ antacids	5-60 min
Esophageal Spasm - associated with cold liquids - improved with nitroglycerin	5-60 min
Peptic Ulcer Disease (PUD) - in the pit of the stomach - worse with meals	5 hours
Gallbladder Disease - Right Upper belly pain or lower chest - in between shoulder blades - worse with meals	hours
Musculoskeletal - worse with movement - local tenderness - worse with pushing on the chest	variable

that time is of the essence. Cardiologists have a saying: "Time is muscle." This means that in the event of a heart attack, the amount of time it takes to get treatment determines the amount of damage to the heart muscle. The longer it takes to receive treatment, the more heart muscle tissue will die and be permanently damaged. The faster you receive treatment, the less damage to the heart muscle and the better your chances of survival.

Knowing the symptoms and warning signs of CHD and heart attack is critical

Reasons People Wait to Call 911

- Embarrassment
- Think they'll look silly
- Denial
- Responsibilities/too busy
- Absence of chest pain
- Blame symptoms on indigestion
- Financial concerns

Surviving a Heart Attack
- Know the symptoms and warning signs.
- Call 911 immediately.
- Chew an aspirin.
- Have family members trained in CPR.
- Take a nitroglycerin tablet (if they have been prescribed to you).

for survival. If you're experiencing any symptoms associated with heart attack, call 911 immediately. Far too many people delay calling for help. I've heard every excuse possible from my patients who have had heart attacks but waited to call for help. Some say they felt embarrassed or were afraid of appearing silly. Some were in denial about what was happening to them. Some were so concerned about their many responsibilities—job, family, children, pets, volunteer work—that they thought, "I don't have time to be in the hospital with a heart attack." For some, the absence of crushing chest pain made them doubt that they were actually having a heart attack. Some who had atypical symptoms blamed their discomfort on indigestion and hoped it would just go away. Some people were worried about how much money it would cost to go to the hospital.

I cannot stress enough that if you think you are having a heart attack, call 911 immediately. When you call for help, the 911 operator may recommend that you chew an aspirin while you wait for the ambulance to arrive. Aspirin thins the blood and inhibits platelets from forming blood clots. Chewing the aspirin rather than swallowing it allows it to work faster to thin the blood.

If you have already been diagnosed with CHD, make sure your family is aware of the symptoms and warning signs of a heart attack. Encourage family members to get trained in CPR in case your heart stops due to a heart attack. Talk to your doctor about nitroglycerin tablets to see if you should have them on hand in the event of a heart attack.

CHAPTER 4

GET A DIAGNOSIS

G regory, 45, was in the middle of a meeting at work when he started feeling an unusual pain in his chest. Always health-conscious, he recognized that something wasn't right and made an appointment with me at my office. When he arrived, I asked him about his medical history, and he explained that he had never had any surgeries, major illnesses, or chronic conditions. When I questioned him about his family history, however, he shrugged his shoulders. "I don't know anything about my family history—medical or otherwise," he said. "I was adopted."

Even though Gregory looked healthy and fit, I did an EKG on him. His EKG appeared abnormal, which made me suspect acute coronary syndrome (ACS), so I sent him to the ER. There, he was given an aspirin and had blood drawn, including cardiac biomarkers. His cholesterol levels, including his LP(a), were very high. Considering his young age and the fact that he ate a healthy diet and exercised regularly, this suggested that his condition may have been genetic.

When his cardiac biomarkers were noted as higher than normal, suggesting that his heart wasn't getting enough blood, Gregory was admitted to the hospital for monitoring and given nitroglycerin and intravenous heparin. The following day, Gregory's biomarker levels had increased even more, so he was taken to the cath lab for further evaluation. There we found that his left anterior descending (LAD) artery was about 80 percent blocked.

Gregory's case is typical in that we could tell from the EKG that he had ACS, but it took several tests to accurately diagnose the source of his chest pain. Because those exams helped us pinpoint the problem, we were able to place a stent to open up his artery, and Gregory left the hospital with improved blood flow and a plan for ongoing treatment for his CHD.

Gregory did the right thing in seeking a diagnosis for his chest pain. If you have any of the risk factors or symptoms of CHD, it's important to get a diagnosis. A rapid diagnosis can lead to treatment of CHD, which may slow or even reverse atherosclerosis and may help you avoid a heart attack. In the case of a heart attack, early treatment can minimize damage to the heart muscle and in some cases, can mean the difference between life and death.

Diagnosing CHD, ACS, and in particular a heart attack can be a complicated process, in part because many of the symptoms are also associated with other conditions. In addition, there isn't one definitive test that will determine if you have CHD or that you're having a heart attack. Whether you are in the ER with symptoms of a possible heart attack or at an office visit with a cardiologist, doctors will use a wide variety of screening tools and tests to evaluate the health of your heart.

WHAT IS A CARDIOLOGIST?

To get a diagnosis for CHD or for follow-up appointments after a heart attack, ACS episode, or bypass surgery, you will see a cardiologist. A cardiologist is a medical doctor who specializes in treating diseases of the heart and circulatory system. To become a cardiologist, a person needs to go through rigorous training. After graduating medical school, cardiology candidates must complete a three-year residency in internal medicine followed by a fellow-ship in general or interventional cardiology that may last three to five years.

Most cardiologists are members or fellows of the American College of Cardiology (ACC). Interventional cardiologists may also become members of the Society for Cardiac Angiography and Interventions (SCAI).

Many physicians and cardiologists in the U.S. are graduates of foreign medical schools. For foreign medical school graduates to become physicians in the U.S., they must have graduated from a medical school that is recognized by the World Health Organization and the American Medical Association. These foreign medical school graduates are required to take an entrance exam administered by the National Board of Medical Examiners and must achieve scores higher than their respective U.S. medical school graduates. After passing the exam, they must go through the same application process for residency and fellowship programs.

All doctors in the U.S. must pass the U.S. Medical Licensing Examination (USMLE) to obtain a medical license. The USMLE is a three-part test that assesses a physician's knowledge as well as their ability to speak and understand English and to communicate with patients. All cardiologists must maintain board certification in internal medicine, cardiology, and their particular subspecialty, such as interventional cardiology. You can verify a cardiologist's certification by entering their name on the American Board of Internal Medicine's website (http://www.abim.org/verify-physician.aspx).

MEETING WITH A CARDIOLOGIST

CHD is an elusive disease. If you have stable angina, you can make an appointment to see a cardiologist or primary care physician for evaluation. If you are experiencing chest pain with some symptoms described above that suggest unstable angina, however, you need to seek immediate attention in an emergency department. Remember, if you suspect you are having a heart attack, call 911.

Many people feel overwhelmed the first time they visit a cardiologist. You may be unsure about what to expect from your appointment or worried that you'll get a bad diagnosis. By familiarizing yourself with the process, you may feel more at ease about your visit. To make the most of your time with the cardiologist or emergency physician, bring the following items with you to your appointment:

- A list of medications and the dosages you are taking (or bring the medications with you)
- A list of over-the-counter drugs, vitamins, and supplements you are taking
- A list of past surgical procedures
- A list of any health conditions
- A list of any major health conditions among close family members
- Copies of your most recent lab results
- A list of your healthcare providers
- A list of questions you want to ask

MEDICAL HISTORY AND FAMILY HISTORY

Typically, your cardiologist will review your medical history and ask about any family history of heart disease. Expect to answer questions about any health issues or surgeries in your past or that close family members have experienced. Your doctor will also ask you about any previous heart attacks, strokes, chest pain, or shortness of breath. Be prepared to describe any symptoms you have experienced. Your doctor may ask you the following questions about your symptoms:

- How long do the symptoms last?
- How often do you experience the symptoms?
- How long have you been having the symptoms?
- What triggers the symptoms?
- What, if anything, worsens the symptoms?
- What, if anything, relieves the symptoms?

In addition to asking about your medical history and symptoms, your doctor will likely ask you about the following lifestyle factors:

- History of smoking
- Drinking habits
- Diet
- Exercise routines
- Mental stress levels

PHYSICAL EXAM

As part of your visit, your doctor will conduct a physical exam. This is an opportunity for your physician to check your general appearance and vital signs, including your blood pressure, heart rate, and breathing rate. In addition, you can expect your physician to listen to your heart, lungs, and gastrointestinal system with a stethoscope. This routine exam allows your doctor to detect abnormal heart sounds, such as an irregular heartbeat or a heart murmur, which may result from damage to the heart muscle or valves due to poor circulation.

ELECTROCARDIOGRAM (EKG)

Your physician will obtain an electrocardiogram (EKG). This common test records the electrical activity of your heart and can help detect heart problems. An EKG can check your heart rhythm, assess blood flow to your heart, detect a heart attack, identify previous heart attacks, and monitor for other issues.

This simple, noninvasive test is painless and takes about 10 minutes. A number of electrodes with adhesive pads will be placed at various points on your chest and possibly on your arms and legs. Wires from the electrodes attach to the EKG computer, which creates a graph of your heart's electrical impulses. During the test, you simply lie quietly while the machine does the work. When the test is complete, the electrodes are removed.

Your doctor will review your results with you. A normal EKG doesn't necessarily rule out CHD. You could have some narrowing of the arteries that doesn't show on the EKG. An abnormal EKG can be an indicator of:

Abnormal heart rate: An EKG can determine if your heart is beating too fast (tachycardia) or too slow (bradycardia). A normal heart rate is between 60 and 100 beats per minute.

Abnormal heart rhythm: The heart typically beats in a rhythmic pattern. An EKG can show if your heart is beating in a nonrhythmic fashion.

Heart attack: An EKG can immediately detect a heart attack and can help determine what type of heart attack a person is having. A pattern known as ST-elevation indicates a complete blockage of an artery. This is called a STEMI (ST-segment elevated myocardial infarction) heart attack. If there is no sign of ST-elevation, but other tests indicate a heart attack, it is called an NSTEMI (non-ST-segment elevation myocardial infarction). In the event of a heart attack, a series of EKG tests will be conducted to evaluate changes in your heart's electrical activity in response to treatment.

BLOOD TESTS

If you're complaining of chest pain or other heart attack symptoms, a number of blood tests, known as cardiac biomarkers, may be ordered. These biomarkers can detect damage to the heart muscle. To make a proper diagnosis, doctors will evaluate blood test results along with your medical history and EKG findings.

Troponin: Troponin is a protein released in the heart muscle in response to heart damage. Elevated troponin levels are a strong indicator of ACS and, specifically, a heart attack. However, troponin levels may be high for other reasons. For example, people with diabetes, heart failure, kidney problems, or lung clots may have above normal troponin levels.

Creatine kinase and CK-MB: Creatine kinase is an enzyme that plays a role in muscle function. When levels of the enzyme are elevated, it indicates muscle damage and may point to a heart attack. CK-MB is an isoenzyme that increases due to damage to the heart muscle. It is normally present only in trace amounts in the blood or may even be undetectable, but levels rise following a heart attack. These two blood tests were once the most common labs used to diagnose a heart attack; however, troponin is now the preferred blood testing method.

STRESS TEST

A stress test, or treadmill test, assesses your heart's activity while exercising. This noninvasive test is generally performed while you walk on a treadmill or ride a stationary bike. Typically, you start on a flat level on the treadmill or at a low level of resistance on the bike. The test gets increasingly difficult as you go, requiring more effort from you. The grade of the treadmill may be raised so you are walking uphill, or the tension on the stationary bike may get higher, requiring you to pedal harder.

As you exert yourself, your heart requires more blood and oxygen, so it has to work harder. This causes your heart rate to rise, which helps cardiologists detect problems with how your heart muscle functions. You are hooked up to an EKG, which measures your heart's electrical activity, as you perform the test. Your blood pressure and heart rate are also monitored throughout the test. If at any time you feel chest pain, shortness of breath, or dizziness, you may stop the test.

A stress test can be used to detect:

- poor circulation
- inadequate blood supply in the coronary arteries
- irregular heartbeat
- whether your heart medicine is working adequately
- whether you require additional testing or treatment

A stress test takes about an hour. The exercise portion lasts only about 15 minutes, but preparation before the test and monitoring after the test adds another 45 minutes. To prepare for a stress test:

- Avoid eating or drinking anything other than water for two to four hours prior to testing.
- Ask your doctor if you should stop taking any of your usual medications, vitamins, or supplements.
- Wear comfortable clothing and walking shoes with a rubber sole.

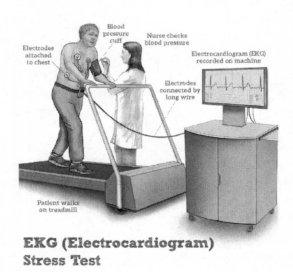

EKG (Electrocardiogram) Stress Test

NUCLEAR STRESS TEST

Your doctor may suggest a nuclear stress test in some cases, such as when your simple stress test produces inconclusive results. This test measures blood flow to your heart while you are at rest and also while your heart is stressed. A scanner is used to take two sets of images: One set is taken at rest and another is taken while your heart is working harder.

For this test, a radioactive dye called a nuclear isotope, such as thallium or technitium, is injected into one of your veins. While you are lying down, a special camera will take images that show how the nuclear isotope moves through your body to your heart. Then you'll be asked to repeat the exercise portion of your stress test. When your heart is pumping at maximum capacity, another dose of the nuclear isotope will be injected, and more images of your heart will be captured. If you aren't able to exercise for any reason, medicine will be injected that causes your heart to pump faster, similar to the way it would during exercise.

A nuclear stress test can detect all the same issues that a simple stress test can show. In addition, its images can reveal both live and dead tissues in the heart, helping your doctor diagnose any damage from a previous heart attack. Normal results from a nuclear stress test indicate that blood is likely flowing adequately though your coronary arteries. Abnormal results may indicate reduced blood flow to the heart due to narrowing of the arteries or a blockage in one of your arteries.

ECHOCARDIOGRAM

An echocardiogram, or "echo," is a test that uses ultrasound to create images of your heart as it beats and pumps blood. An echo produces images of the heart's chambers, valves, and walls in addition to the blood vessels that feed and branch off from the heart. These images can help a doctor diagnose:

- heart attack or previous heart attack
- coronary artery disease
- inflammation of the pericardium (the sac surrounding the heart)
- valve problems
- lung clots
- diseases involving the aorta
- complications from heart attack
- rupture of the heart muscle
- fluid around the heart or a leak in the heart valve

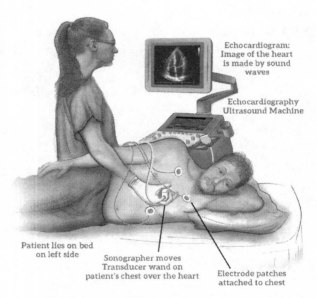

Echocardiogram: Image of the heart is made by sound waves

Echocardiography Ultrasound Machine

Patient lies on bed on left side

Sonographer moves Transducer wand on patient's chest over the heart

Electrode patches attached to chest

Echocardiogram
Ultrasound of the Heart

An echocardiogram is a noninvasive, painless test. It can be done in your cardiologist's office, in a lab, or in the hospital. For this test, electrodes will be placed on your chest and attached to an EKG machine to monitor your heart's electrical activity. A special gel that helps transmit sound waves will be applied to your chest. A small, plastic, hand-held probe called a transducer will be passed back and forth over your chest, sending out sound waves and receiving the "echo" from sound waves that bounce off your heart back to the transducer. These sound waves are transformed into images displayed on a video monitor for your doctor to review. In many cases, your doctor will show you the images so you can see your heart as it beats.

Your doctor will take your echo test results into consideration along with your medical history and other diagnostic test results to form a diagnosis.

COMPUTED TOMOGRAPHY ANGIOGRAM (CTA)

A computed tomography angiogram (CTA) scan is a minimally invasive test that uses X-rays to examine blood flow in the coronary arteries. While typical X-rays take two-dimensional pictures of the body's bones, CT scans offer a much more detailed cross-sectional view of the body, showing not only bones but also blood vessels. This is very helpful for diagnosing CHD because CTA scans reveal any plaque buildup, calcification, narrowing, or blockages in the arteries.

For this test, you'll lie on a table that passes through the opening of a doughnut-shaped scanner. Iodine, which is a contrast dye, is administered into a vein in your arm or hand. The contrast dye causes your blood vessels to show up in a more pronounced fashion in the resulting images, making it easier for doctors to evaluate how blood is flowing through your arteries. You'll be given a special medicine called a beta blocker to slow your heart rate to between 60 to 70 beats per minute, which allows the scanner to obtain clearer images of your heart and its arteries. Typically, you need to hold your breath for at least five seconds as your body passes through the scanner. The procedure usually takes 30 minutes to an hour.

One of the most powerful diagnostic imaging tools available to cardiologists is the 64-slice CT scanner. This device is optimal for visualizing a beating heart because it captures images at a much higher rate than traditional CT scanners. With this scanner, your cardiologist can distinguish whether the cause of your chest discomfort comes from coronary artery disease, a blood clot in the lungs, or a tear in the aorta (aortic dissection).

If there is severe calcium buildup in your coronary arteries, the doctor may have difficulty diagnosing CHD with CTA scanning, especially in smaller arteries. The calcium buildup may show narrowing in an artery when there isn't or, vice-versa, may indicate that arteries look healthy when they are not. The medical community continues to make advances in CTA scanning technology, however, which should improve this capability in the future.

If your doctor tells you that your CTA scan results are normal, it means:

- blood flow in your arteries is normal
- there is no evidence of narrowed arteries
- there is no evidence of blocked arteries
- there is no evidence of plaque buildup
- there is no sign of an aortic aneurysm or aortic dissection

If your test results are abnormal, it may mean that:

- one or more arteries are blocked or partially blocked
- a blood clot is reducing blood flow
- a plaque is reducing blood flow
- an aortic aneurysm or aortic dissection is present

Based on your results, your cardiologist may recommend other testing or treatment. Rest assured that CTA scanning poses minimal risks. The level of radiation from a CTA scan is considered safe and in the rare event that you have an allergic reaction to the contrast dye, it can be relieved with medication.

CORONARY MRI

A coronary MRI, also called a cardiac MRI, is a minimally invasive diagnostic imaging test that uses magnets and radio waves to produce images of your heart. Images from a coronary MRI can help your doctor diagnose CHD or damage from a previous heart attack, as well as other heart-related issues.

For this test, you'll be required to lie very still on a table that is inserted into a tunnel-like machine. Inside the machine, you'll hear loud buzzing and clanking as it takes images of your heart. If you have a fear of being in tight, cramped places, you may want to ask your doctor to prescribe a mild sedative that you can take prior to your test. If you take a sedative, be sure to have a friend or family member available to drive you home after your coronary MRI.

There are advantages and disadvantages of coronary MRI compared with CTA scanning. On the plus side, coronary MRI involves no radiation, doesn't require any contrast dye, and doesn't need medication to slow your heart rate. It may also provide more accurate results for people who have severe calcification of the arteries. On the downside, the images it produces are not as precise as the pictures from coronary CTA. In addition, if you have a pacemaker or an implanted medical device, you can't undergo a coronary MRI.

MYOCARDIAL PERFUSION IMAGING (MPI)

Myocardial perfusion imaging (MPI) is a noninvasive scan that evaluates blood flow to the heart muscle. This test evaluates how well your heart is pumping and can detect if there are any parts of your heart that aren't receiving adequate amounts of blood. A doctor may order an MPI test to help determine whether chest pain is due to narrowed or blocked arteries. By reviewing the blood flow within the heart muscle, your doctor can diagnose if any coronary arteries are blocked. If you've had a previous heart attack, even a silent ischemia, it will show up on an MPI test.

If your MPI results are normal, it is a good sign that any chest discomfort you're experiencing is due to something other than your heart or coronary arteries. If your results are abnormal or if they reveal blockages, your cardiologist may recommend further treatment, such as a coronary angiogram.

CORONARY ANGIOGRAPHY

A coronary angiogram, which uses special X-ray imaging to see your heart's blood vessels, is considered the gold standard of diagnostic tests for detecting arterial blockages. This imaging test usually isn't ordered until after other noninvasive tests—such as EKG, stress test, or echocardiogram—have been performed. With imaging from an angiogram, your doctor can see how blood is flowing through your arteries and within the heart muscle. An angiogram can:

- detect how many of your arteries have narrowing or blockages
- identify where narrowing and blockages are within your arteries
- show how much narrowing or blockage there is

Thanks to advances in cardiology, doctors may be able to treat any narrowing or blockages with procedures, such as angioplasty or stenting, immediately after diagnosis. (See more about these procedures in Chapter 6.)

Coronary angiogram, which involves cardiac catheterization, is typically performed in a hospital setting. Prior to your procedure, you'll be given a sedative that will relax you but will allow you to remain awake. During catheterization, a long, thin plastic tube called a catheter is inserted into an artery in your groin or in your arm. The catheter is threaded through the blood vessel to the coronary arteries. Then a contrast dye is injected into the catheter to make the blood vessels and heart more visible in the images produced. A series of X-rays are taken as the dye makes its way to your heart.

These images are displayed on a video screen that allows your cardiologist to see your heart and arteries in action. Doctors can immediately see if an artery is completely blocked or only partially occluded. Cardiologists consider coronary angiography the optimal tool for diagnosing atherosclerosis because it provides a clear view of narrowing and blockages and allows them to pinpoint where the problem areas are within the arteries. They can also visualize how well the blood vessels fill up with blood. In people with blood clots, the blood vessels don't fill up as well. No other diagnostic tool offers such an immediate and precise diagnosis.

If you're in the ER with symptoms of ACS, cardiac catheterization and angiography will be performed on an emergency basis. In other cases, it is scheduled in advance. Your doctor will give you instructions detailing how to prepare for the procedure and what to expect. Routine guidelines for this procedure are:

- Don't eat or drink anything after midnight the night before your angiogram.
- Check with your doctor to see if you should stop taking any of your medications, vitamins, or supplements.
- Tell your doctor if you are allergic to any medicines or if

you have ever had an allergic reaction to contrast dye. Doctors can use medicines prior to the procedure to minimize the chance of an allergic reaction.

- Inform your doctor if you're pregnant.

At the hospital, you will receive a sedative by IV to help you relax. Your vital signs—including your blood pressure and heart rate—will be monitored throughout the procedure. The doctor will make a small incision in your groin or arm to insert the catheter, which will then be threaded to your heart. You may feel some pressure, but it shouldn't be painful. Let your doctor know if you are feeling any discomfort or chest pain. With the catheter in place, a contrast dye will be injected through the tube.

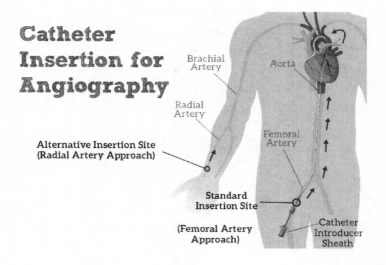

During cardiac catheterization, your cardiologist may perform additional diagnostic imaging tests, such as intravascular ultrasound and optical coherence tomography.

Intravascular ultrasound: This test uses sound waves inside the blood vessels to evaluate the health of your coronary artery walls. It can show whether there is any buildup of plaque on artery walls. To perform this test, a tiny ultrasound wand is inserted into an artery in the groin area and then advanced to your heart. The sound waves are translated into images that can be viewed on a video screen. This diagnostic test is usually performed during another procedure, such as an angiogram.

Optical coherence tomography: Optical coherence tomography (OCT) uses near-infrared light to produce high-resolution images of the blood vessels. OCT allows your cardiologist to view the inner walls of your arteries at 10 times the magnification of intravascular ultrasound. OCT offers clear images of plaque formations on artery walls and assists your cardiologist in taking measurements for stent placement.

Based on the findings of your angiogram, your doctor may perform additional procedures, such as angioplasty or stenting, while you are in the cath lab. You can read more about these procedures in Chapter 6.

When your procedure is complete, the catheter will be removed and the incision area closed. You will be taken to a recovery area where you will need to lie flat for several hours to prevent bleeding. Healthcare professionals will continue to monitor your condition until they deem it is safe for you to return home. Before you leave the hospital, your doctor will go over your results with you and will also provide you with some post-procedure instructions. General guidelines following cardiac catheterization are:

- Drink plenty of fluids to help flush out the contrast dye from your system.
- Avoid strenuous activity for a few days.
- Ask your doctor when you can resume taking your daily

medications, vitamins, and supplements.

- Ask your doctor when you can take a shower or bath.
- Call your doctor if the leg or arm used for the procedure feels cool to the touch, changes color, or feels numb.
- Call your doctor if you notice any bleeding, redness, swelling, drainage, or increased pain at the insertion site.
- If the insertion site will not stop bleeding, call 911.

It's important to understand the risks involved in any procedure. Cardiac catheterization involves some risks, such as exposure to radiation and possible allergic reaction to the contrast dye. Serious risks are rare but include injury to the catheterized artery, irregular heartbeat, kidney damage, infection, stroke, and heart attack.

DEALING WITH YOUR DIAGNOSIS

When you're diagnosed with CHD or you've had a heart attack, it's normal to have an emotional response. You may feel sad, angry, depressed, or anxious about your future. One of the most common responses to a diagnosis of CHD or following a heart attack is depression. In fact, up to 33 percent of people who have a heart attack will experience depression. Not only does depression impact your personal life, relationships, and work, but it also increases your risk of heart attack. Depression can lead to poor lifestyle choices—drinking alcohol and eating junk food, for example—in order to cope. It also has detrimental physiological effects, including increases in stress hormones, cortisol, and glucose levels.

If you are experiencing feelings of sadness, hopelessness, or anxiety that don't go away after several weeks, consider seeing a mental health professional. Ideally, with counseling and treatment, you'll regain your zest for life, which can have a positive impact on your overall heart health.

Part II

TREATING ACUTE CORONARY

SYNDROME

"In my heart there was a kind of fighting that would not let me sleep."
— "Hamlet" by William Shakespeare

CHAPTER 5

MEDICATIONS

J ames, 65, was relaxing at home watching TV when he began experiencing chest pain and shortness of breath. He recognized the symptoms because he had been diagnosed with high cholesterol and CHD about five years earlier and had already undergone bypass surgery to fix blocked arteries. He went straight to the emergency room, fearing he was having a heart attack. In the ER, his EKG didn't detect anything abnormal and his blood biomarker levels were in the normal range. His cholesterol levels, however, were high even though he had been taking cholesterol-lowering medication for several years. James was admitted to the hospital for observation, mainly due to his history of CHD and previous bypass surgery.

As a precaution, I gave James an aspirin and administered a number of other medications that thin the blood, prevent clotting, lower blood pressure, slow the heart rate, and reduce the amount of oxygen the heart requires. These are very powerful treatment options in the case of a heart attack or acute coronary syndrome. About two days later, James' biomarker levels remained normal; however, a nuclear stress test revealed abnormal results, and an angiogram detected a blocked bypass graft. I immediately placed a stent in that clogged bypass graft to improve blood flow, which relieved his chest pain. Thanks to the swift treatment with medications and stent placement, James avoided a possibly deadly heart attack.

In follow-up appointments with James, I advised him to continue taking some of the medications used during his stay as a patient. In addition, because his cholesterol levels had risen, I increased his dosage of cholesterol-lowering medication as a way to reduce the risk of a heart attack in the future.

James is just one of an estimated 5 million to 8 million Americans who head to the ER annually due to chest pain. Approximately 1 million to 2 million of them are diagnosed with acute coronary syndrome (ACS), a broad term describing a variety of conditions related to CHD that require medical attention. Chest pain that occurs suddenly, is severe in nature, or worsens with time is a sign of ACS. Other symptoms of ACS include those associated with possible heart attack, such as shortness of breath, dizziness, perspiration, and nausea. ACS may be due to the following conditions:

Unstable angina: Among individuals with ACS, about 40 percent are diagnosed with unstable angina, which is the acute onset of severe chest pain or angina that doesn't go away after physical exertion.

NSTEMI: About 40 percent of people with ACS are diagnosed with a non-ST-segment elevation myocardial infarction. This type of heart attack typically indicates one or more partial blockages in the arteries.

STEMI: Approximately 20 percent of people with ACS are diagnosed with an ST-segment elevation myocardial infarction, a type of heart attack that is associated with specific EKG changes that are easily recognizable by healthcare professionals. Considered the most dangerous type of heart attack, a STEMI indicates a complete blockage in at least one artery.

Acute Coronary Syndrome (ACS)

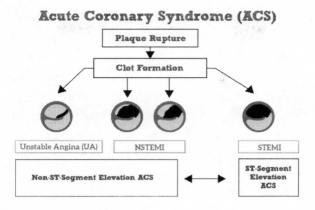

ACS may also encompass sudden cardiac arrest, which occurs when the heart suddenly stops beating. Sometimes due to a heart attack, this life-threatening condition causes a person to fall unconscious—no pulse, no breathing. When 911 is called, EMTs perform lifesaving measures, but they are successful in resuscitating only about 60 percent of people with sudden cardiac arrest. Sadly, the other 40 percent die. The survival rate is higher when CPR is initiated immediately by a family member, friend, or bystander rather than waiting for the arrival of paramedics.

When the lucky ones who are resuscitated arrive at the hospital, they often need emergency measures to lower the risk of dying or brain death. This often involves lowering their body temperature with cooling blankets in the Intensive Care Unit (ICU). These people are also immediately treated with medications and are sent to the cath lab for early invasive treatment.

If you head to the doctor's office or the hospital with chest pain or symptoms of ACS, a healthcare professional will do an initial assessment that includes an EKG. In a doctor's office, if there are signs suggesting ACS, you will be referred to the ER either by ambulance or your own transportation depending on your condition. In a hospital setting, an EKG is usually performed within 10 minutes of your arrival. Your vital signs will also be evaluated, as well as your breathing, oxygen saturation, lipid, and cardiac bio-marker levels.

In all ACS cases, medications are one of the first lines of treatment. Typically, treatment begins with administering a simple aspirin. This is often followed by nitroglycerin or morphine to alleviate chest pain, and blood pressure drugs known as beta blockers. Depending on your condition, the doctor may prescribe a variety of other medications. For some people, noninvasive treatment with medications may be sufficient to alleviate your symptoms and can play a major role in the prevention of a heart attack. In other cases, they may minimize damage to the heart muscle from a heart attack. This chapter details the most commonly used medications to treat ACS.

Some people with ACS may require more invasive treatment. These treatments will be covered in Chapters 6 and 7.

When a Broken Heart Masquerades as ACS
In some cases, symptoms of a heart attack have a completely different cause. Take the case of Joanie Simpson. In 2016, following the death of her beloved Yorkshire terrier, the 61-year-old woke up one morning with severe chest pain. Concerned that she might be having a heart attack, Joanie went to her local ER and was later transported to a major hospital in Houston. An EKG showed ST-elevation, which suggested she might be having a heart attack. Joanie was rushed into the cath lab for coronary angiography. Based on the EKG, doctors expected to find one or more blockages in her arteries. But the angiography revealed that her arteries were clear. Joanie wasn't having a heart attack. Doctors diagnosed her with a far more rare condition: takotsubo cardiomyopathy, which is more commonly referred to as broken-heart syndrome.

First reported in Japan in 1990, broken-heart syndrome almost exclusively affects postmenopausal women between the ages of 58 and 75. In fact, females account for nearly 90 percent of cases. Up to 5 percent of all women who are assessed for heart attack symptoms are diagnosed with broken-heart syndrome. The condition weakens the heart and reduces its ability to squeeze effectively, resulting in pain that mimics symptoms of a heart attack. Treatment for this condition is typically limited to medications, and it usually resolves with time. For Joanie, treatment included the administration of a number of medications that relieved her chest pain and helped heal her broken heart.

Side Effects

Understand that with all medications, there is a possibility of side effects. This chapter describes some of the more common side effects. For a comprehensive list beyond the scope of this book, visit each medication's website.

ANTIPLATELET AGENTS

Aspirin

Aspirin is one of the most commonly used drugs in America. Have a headache? Feel feverish? Have sore joints? Chances are you've popped an aspirin or two for pain relief. Aspirin can also help if you're having chest pain that's related to CHD. Aspirin is an antiplatelet agent that renders platelets inactive. Platelets are blood cells that help your blood to form clots. In everyday life they can be very useful. For example, let's say you slice your hand while preparing dinner and blood starts oozing down your finger. Your body's platelets recognize this and immediately go into action to make the blood clump together to stop the bleeding.

When a blood clot forms in an artery, however, the natural action of platelets can be deadly. Aspirin helps prevent the platelets from forming blood clots, which is important if you have CHD and a possible blockage. If you are at high risk of a heart attack or if you are a heart attack survivor, your doctor may also prescribe that you take a low-dose aspirin daily. In emergency situations, you may be instructed to chew an aspirin, which allows its antiplatelet action to work faster.

Like all drugs, aspirin has side effects. Most commonly, it may cause minor stomach irritation or heartburn.

P2Y12 Inhibitors

Like aspirin, P2Y12 inhibitors are antiplatelet agents that prevent blood from clotting. In some cases, these inhibitors may be prescribed in addition to aspirin to keep platelets from clumping together and to keep blood flowing more efficiently through the blood vessels. If you go to the hospital with chest pain, these drugs are typically administered immediately. If you receive a stent as part of your treatment, you will need to continue taking this medication along with aspirin for at least one year to prevent blockages from forming inside the stent.

Commonly prescribed P2Y12 inhibitors include:

- Clopidogrel (brand name Plavix)
- Prasugrel (brand names Efient and Effient)
- Ticagrelor (brand name Brilinta)

Side effects of these drugs include an increased risk of bleeding and bruising. People taking ticagrelor may experience some shortness of breath, but this usually resolves on its own with time. Because these drugs prevent clotting, it is important to stop taking them about five to seven days prior to any surgical procedure. Ask your doctor for specifics if you take these medications and plan to have surgery.

In rare instances, a person may have a genetic predisposition that prevents these medications from having the desired effect. In these people, a coronary event may occur in spite of taking the drug. If your doctor thinks you may be at high risk of this type of genetic predisposition, a sensitivity test may be performed to see how your body reacts.

ANTICOAGULANTS

Heparin and Enoxaparin

Heparin and enoxaparin (brand name Lovenox) are anticoagulants that are known for their clot-busting capabilities. Not only do they reduce the blood's ability to form clots, but they may also help dissolve existing clots. People who come to the hospital with symptoms of acute coronary syndrome, unstable angina, or heart attack are often given one of these medications. These drugs are usually only administered on a temporary basis. If you undergo stent placement, or if your condition stabilizes, your doctor will generally stop administering anticoagulants.

Side effects associated with anticoagulants include an increased risk of bleeding and a decrease in platelet count. A decrease in platelet count may occur when heparin is administered intravenously and requires discontinuation of the medication and possible treatment. These medications may interact with other drugs, so be sure to inform your doctor of all medications you're taking.

ANTIANGINAL AGENTS

Nitrates

If you're experiencing acute angina in the hospital or if you have recurring but stable chest pain, your doctor may prescribe

Nitroglycerin's Explosive History

You may be surprised to learn that nitroglycerin is an active ingredient in dynamite. How did this explosive substance become one of the leading treatments for relieving angina? In the 1860s, workers in dynamite factories found that coming in contact with nitroglycerin seemed to relieve their chest pain. Around the same time, people in the medical community began experimenting with nitrates as a possible treatment for angina. By the 1870s, scientists discovered that using a very small amount of nitroglycerin diluted with other substances rendered it safe as a treatment for chest pain.

nitrates in the form of nitroglycerin. Nitroglycerin is a fast-acting drug that can provide quick relief from chest pain. This medication is a vasodilator, which means it dilates the arteries and other blood vessels. When blood vessels are widened, blood flows more easily to the heart. This increases the amount of oxygen reaching the heart while decreasing the workload on the heart.

Nitroglycerin is usually prescribed as tablets or a spray that you put under your tongue. In some cases of extreme chest pain in the ER, however, it may be administered intravenously. This usually relieves chest pain quickly.

If you are self-administering nitroglycerin for chest pain related to coronary artery disease and it doesn't resolve your chest pain immediately, doses can be administered every two to five minutes apart—up to three doses. If your chest pain is not relieved after three doses, go to the ER.

It's important to be aware of the side effects associated with nitroglycerin. The most troublesome side effect of taking nitroglycerin is that it can lower blood pressure, making you feel dizzy or lightheaded. Never take nitroglycerin if you take medications for erectile dysfunction, as this can reduce blood pressure to dangerously low levels.

Beta Blockers

Beta blockers, also referred to as beta-adrenergic blocking agents, are often prescribed to treat chest pain. These drugs lower heart rate and reduce the heart's oxygen requirement. This allows the heart to pump with less force. Beta blockers widen blood vessels to improve blood flow, which reduces blood pressure. These combined actions can be extremely helpful in alleviating angina.

If a person comes to the hospital with chest pain, we usually administer beta blockers within the first 24 hours. Research has shown that heart attack patients who receive treatment with beta blockers in the hospital are at a reduced risk of dying after being discharged. These drugs are so beneficial, doctors recommend you continue to use them for at least three years and sometimes even longer periods of time after a heart attack.

Commonly prescribed beta blockers include:

- Metoprolol (brand name Toprol)
- Atenolol (brand name Tenormin)
- Carvedilol (brand name Coreg)
- Labetalol (brand name Trandate)

The most common side effects of beta blockers include fatigue, cold hands and feet, and weight gain. Other less common side effects include depression, shortness of breath, and sleep disturbances. Beta blockers have also been known to increase triglycerides and decrease HDL "good" cholesterol, so your doctor will need to monitor your lipids and treat any irregularities as needed.

Beta blockers are not recommended for people who have an abnormally low resting heart rate or who are allergic to beta blockers. They are not advised for people with asthma because they may trigger an asthma attack. If you have diabetes, exercise caution when taking beta blockers. These drugs may mask some of the symptoms associated with low blood sugar levels in people with diabetes, such as a fast heartbeat, sweating, lightheadedness, and feelings of anxiety. Because of this, be sure to discuss your condition with your doctor.

Calcium Channel Blockers

Calcium channel blockers are often used to treat chest pain. As you might suspect, they work by blocking calcium from entering the cells within the heart and in the blood vessels. This relaxes the arteries, allowing blood to flow more freely to the heart muscle. In turn, this lowers blood pressure and reduces the force with which the heart has to pump. In some cases, it may also normalize an irregular heartbeat.

Commonly prescribed calcium channel blockers include:

- Diltiazem (brand names Cardizem, Tiazac, and others)
- Verapamil (brand names Calan and Verelan)
- Amlodipine (brand name Norvasc)

Note that nifedipine (brand names Adalat CC, Afeditab CR, and Procardia) is typically avoided in people with acute coronary syndrome or heart attack because it can increase heart rate.

The most common side effects of calcium channel blockers include constipation, headaches, dizziness, allergic reactions, drowsiness, nausea, flushing, and swelling of the hands. While taking calcium channel blockers, it is important to avoid drinking grapefruit juice because it may increase the severity of side effects.

Ranolazine

If you continue to have chest pain despite the use of other therapies, your doctor may add ranolazine (brand name Ranexa) to your treatment plan. This medication improves cardiac function without reducing blood pressure. Avoid drinking grapefruit juice or eating grapefruit while taking this medication. Side effects include headaches, nausea, dizziness, and constipation.

BLOOD PRESSURE MEDICATIONS

ACE Inhibitors

Angiotensin converting enzyme (ACE) inhibitors are drugs that prevent the formation of angiotensin, a substance that narrows blood vessels. Angiotensin increases blood pressure and forces the heart to work harder. By blocking angiotensin, ACE drugs produce the opposite effect: lowering blood pressure and reducing the heart's workload. This improves blood flow in people with poor coronary circulation. ACE inhibitors have been proven very effective in healing damage to the heart muscle after a heart attack. It also aids in improving the heart's ability to contract in people whose heart does not squeeze tightly enough.

If you go to the hospital with chest pain, these drugs are often prescribed about 36 to 48 hours prior to being discharged.

Commonly prescribed ACE inhibitors include:

- Lisinopril (brand names Prinivil and Zestril)
- Benazepril (brand name Lotensin)
- Enalapril (brand name Vasotec)
- Captopril
- Ramipril (brand name Altace)

As with any drug, ACE inhibitors have side effects. The most common side effect is a dry cough, which occurs in approximately 10 percent of people taking the drug. Other side effects include headaches, dizziness, fatigue, loss of taste, and increased potassium levels. As a safeguard, your doctor will monitor your potassium levels while you are taking ACE inhibitors.

ARBs

Similar to ACE inhibitors, angiotensin II receptor blockers (ARBs) block the action of angiotensin, the substance that causes blood vessels to narrow. ARBs widen blood vessels to allow improved blood flow and lower blood pressure. ARBs may be prescribed if you are not able to take ACE inhibitors for any reason. Like ARBs, they may not be administered immediately if you go to the hospital with chest pain, but they are likely to be prescribed prior to being discharged from the hospital.

Commonly prescribed ARBs include:

- Losartan (brand name Cozaar)
- Valsartan (brand name Diovan)
- Candesartan (brand name Atacand)

ARBs have many of the same side effects as ACE inhibitors, including dry cough (although it is rare with ARBs), headaches, dizziness, fatigue, loss of taste, and increased potassium levels. Your doctor will monitor your potassium levels while you are taking ARBs.

Clonidine

Clonidine works in the brain as a nerve inhibitor. When this drug is administered, your brain sends messages to the nerves in your blood vessels instructing them to relax. This lowers blood pressure and may reduce heart rate. Clonidine, which can be taken orally or topically as a patch, may be prescribed if other blood pressure medicines do not control your symptoms. Catapres is the most commonly prescribed brand.

Side effects include fatigue, dry mouth, constipation, dry eyes, sleep problems, and dizziness. It's important that you don't stop taking clonidine abruptly, as this can cause blood pressure to rebound and shoot up to dangerous levels.

Hydralazine

Hydralazine is a vasodilator that relaxes the blood vessels to lower blood pressure. In emergency situations, this drug may be given orally or intravenously to improve blood flow. Apresoline is the most commonly prescribed brand.

Side effects include headache, flushing, upset stomach, diarrhea, and stuffy nose.

THROMBOLYTIC THERAPY

Thrombolytic medication, also known as fibrinolytic therapy, works to break up and dissolve blood clots. The most commonly used thrombolytic is called tissue plasminogen activator (tPA). These drugs must be delivered within the first 24 hours of the onset of a heart attack, and the sooner they are given, the more effective they are. They can restore blood flow and reduce damage due to a heart attack. Thrombolytics are typically used in conjunction with other medications, including blood thinners such as heparin or lovenox, aspirin, P2Y12 inhibitors, and anticoagulants. These powerful clot busters reduce complications from heart attack and reduce the risk of dying.

The most common side effect associated with thrombolytics is bleeding.

PAIN RELIEVERS

Morphine

In some instances in a hospital setting, small doses of morphine may be used to control pain from angina. Morphine causes relaxation of the heart muscle and arteries, reduces the need for oxygen, and decreases the overall workload on the heart. In the hospital, morphine is usually administered intravenously.

You may associate morphine with drug addiction, but be aware that in general, this drug is only administered in the hospital, in very small doses, and for a limited period of time. You can rest assured that this eliminates any possibility of addiction.

CHOLESTEROL MEDICATIONS

Statins

Statins are cholesterol-lowering medications that can reduce the risk of heart attack, stroke, and death from CHD by up to 35 percent. In people who have already had a heart attack, taking statins can reduce the risk of another heart attack by up to 40 percent. This medication works by blocking enzymes in the liver that produce cholesterol. Research shows that these drugs are effective in lowering LDL "bad" cholesterol. They may also lower triglycerides and LP(a) and can increase HDL "good" cholesterol. In some cases, statins may help in the reabsorption of cholesterol in plaque buildups, effectively reducing the size of a plaque.

Introduced in the 1980s, statins have become one of the most commonly prescribed class of drugs in America. In fact, nearly 29 percent of all adults over age 40 use prescription cholesterol-lowering medication, according to the Centers for Disease Control and Prevention (CDC). Statins are typically prescribed for the ongoing management of cholesterol levels. They are not commonly used as an emergency treatment.

Should you take statins? It depends on your medical history, cholesterol levels, and additional risk factors. Statins are typically recommended if you meet any of the following criteria:

- You have been diagnosed with CHD.
- You have a history of stroke or peripheral artery disease.
- Your LDL is 160 mg/dl or higher.
- You are 40 to 75 years old with a history of high cholesterol and at least one other risk factor for CHD family history, diabetes, high blood pressure, or history of smoking).

Commonly prescribed statins include:

- Lovastatin (brand names Mevacor and Altoprev)
- Atorvastatin (brand name Lipitor)
- Simvastatin (brand name Zocor)
- Rosuvastatin (brand name Crestor)
- Pravastatin (brand name Pravachol)

Some of the more common side effects seen with statins include muscle pain, achiness, soreness, and weakness. If you feel like you are experiencing weakness, your doctor can perform some simple tests to assess your condition. In rare cases, taking these medications may cause muscle or liver damage. Because of this, your doctor will monitor your liver function on a regular basis. Some people may experience an increase in blood sugar levels, so it's important for your doctor to check your levels on a regular basis. Symptoms of memory loss have also been reported. If you notice any changes in your memory, see your doctor for an evaluation.

In general, those who are more likely to experience side effects while taking statins include:

- women
- senior citizens

- people taking multiple medications
- people with kidney or liver disease
- moderate to heavy drinkers

Bile Acid Binding Resins

People with high levels of LDL cholesterol who are unable to take statins may be prescribed medications called bile acid binding resins. Bile acid is produced in the liver in a process that involves converting cholesterol into bile acid. These drugs remove bile acid from the liver by sending it to the intestines where it is then excreted in the stool. This forces the liver to create more bile acid, which requires the conversion of more cholesterol. Ultimately, as more cholesterol is used to produce bile acid, lower levels of LDL cholesterol remain in the bloodstream.

In general, these drugs are not as effective at lowering cholesterol as statins. They typically result in only a mild to moderate decrease in LDL levels. To improve their effectiveness, they may be used in conjunction with other medications. However, these drugs should not be taken at the same time as other medications. It is advised to wait four hours either before or after taking other medications.

Commonly prescribed bile acid binding resins include:

- Colesevelam (brand name Welchol)
- Cholestyramine (brand names Questran and Prevalite)
- Colestipol (brand name Colestid)

Side effects associated with bile acid binding resins include constipation, stomachache, headache, muscle pain, and flu-like symptoms.

Ezetimibe

Another type of medication called ezetimibe (brand name Zetia) aims to lower cholesterol levels by reducing the amount of cholesterol absorbed from food. The reduction in cholesterol levels is not as strong with this drug compared to statins. In some cases, when statins do not lower cholesterol levels enough, ezetimibe may be added.

Side effects include stomachache, nausea, and vomiting. In people with liver disease, there is a risk of liver damage, especially if you are also taking statins.

Fibrates

Fibric acid derivatives known as fibrates can lower triglyceride levels and may increase HDL cholesterol, but are generally ineffective at lowering LDL cholesterol. If you have very high triglyceride levels—over 1000—you may benefit from taking fibrates. These drugs may be combined with statins to help lower LDL levels.

Commonly prescribed fibrates include:

- Fenofibrate (brand names Antara, Lipofen, Tricor, and Triglide)
- Gemfibrozil (brand name Lopid)

Side effects include stomachache, nausea, gas, heartburn, and rash.

Niacin

Niacin, which is commonly known as vitamin B3, may be recommended to raise HDL and lower triglyceride levels. The mechanism behind this action remains unknown, but some medical experts believe it stops the release of fatty acids into the bloodstream. Niacin is only effective in high doses and even then, the results are mild to moderate. It is often prescribed in conjunction with statins. Niaspan is the most commonly prescribed brand of niacin. This drug should be taken at night after a small fatty snack.

Side effects include flushing, itching, sweating, and tingling. You can decrease the risk of symptoms by avoiding spicy foods, alcohol, and hot beverages.

PCSK9 Inhibitors

Newer lines of defense against high cholesterol are medications known as PCSK9 inhibitors. Approved in 2015, these powerful agents are available only in an injectable form and have been shown to lower LDL cholesterol by as much as 60 percent when taken in conjunction with statins. These drugs are administered with a pen-like injector one to two times per month. Currently, the cost associated with these new drugs—about $14,000 per year—puts them out of reach of many people who could benefit from them. However, costs will likely come down with time.

These biologic drugs, known as monoclonal antibodies, work by blocking a protein called proprotein convertase subtilisin kexin 9 (PCSK9) in the liver. Inactivating PCSK9 allows the body to move LDL out of the bloodstream, resulting in lower LDL levels.

Commonly prescribed PCSK9 inhibitors include:

- Alirocumab (brand name Praluent)
- Evolocumab (brand name Repatha)

Side effects include flu-like symptoms and reactions at the injection site.

MEDICATIONS TO TREAT COMPLICATIONS FROM ACS

Having ACS can lead to complications. For example, about 20 percent of people who are diagnosed with unstable angina or NSTEMI will also develop some form of heart arrhythmia. Medical experts believe this occurs due to increased stress hormones as a result of the heart working too hard. Arrhythmia may lead to other complications, including inflammation of the pericardium (the sac surrounding the heart), electrolyte abnormalities, and oxygen deprivation (known as hypoxia). An irregular heartbeat can be life threatening, but in most cases, rhythm disorders can be treated with blood thinners and antiarrhythmic drugs.

The most commonly prescribed antiarrhythmic medications include:

- Amiodarone (brand name Cordarone)
- Flecainide (brand name Tambocor)
- Procainamide (brand name Procanbid)
- Sotalol (brand name Betapace)

Side effects associated with these drugs include lightheadedness, dizziness, fainting, cough, loss of appetite, changes in taste, diarrhea or constipation, and increased sensitivity to sunlight. In addition to medications, a pacemaker may be used temporarily in the initial stages of arrhythmia or other heartbeat issues. It is removed after healthy circulation and heart rhythm have been restored.

CHAPTER 6

ANGIOPLASTY AND STENTS

Miguel, 58, woke up one morning with severe pain in his chest. He nudged his wife, Gina, and told her how bad he felt. She didn't want to take any chances, so she called 911. Before the paramedics arrived, Miguel lost consciousness and stopped breathing. Gina was terrified and confused. Her husband, who worked for a major airline in the Houston area, was healthy and in good shape. Sure, he had high blood pressure, but he took medication for it, watched what he ate, and exercised regularly. How could he be having a heart attack, she wondered. Within 10 minutes of calling for help, the EMTs arrived. They shocked Miguel's heart and performed CPR, successfully resuscitating him. As they were en route to the hospital where I was on call, they performed an EKG, transmitted the results showing ACS, and informed us Miguel had passed out—"coded," in doctor speak—and had been revived.

I went into action to prepare for his arrival. Miguel was conscious when he was wheeled in to the ER, but his blood pressure was very low. Within 30 minutes, Miguel was in the cath lab, where I found a major blockage in his left anterior descending artery, the widowmaker. Working quickly, I placed a stent in the clogged artery and positioned a balloon pump in the aorta to help his heart pump blood. With these in place, his condition improved and he was out of danger. Miguel stayed in the hospital for about three days before going home. Gina couldn't thank me enough. When Miguel had passed out at home, she thought he was going to die.

Today, Miguel's heart function is normal. He's back to work at the airline, exercising, and coming to my office for regular follow-up visits. With routine checkups, we can catch any changes in his heart health early.

Miguel was in a life-or-death situation when we made the decision to use invasive techniques to treat him. But you don't have to be unconscious or have a major blockage in the widowmaker artery to warrant treatment with invasive procedures. Depending on your condition and your response to treatment with medications, your doctor may recommend more invasive procedures, such as angiography, catheterization, stent or balloon placement, or even bypass surgery.

In general, people with ACS are more likely to be treated with some form of invasive procedure now than in the past. This is because research has shown that these interventional procedures reduce death rates and decrease the incidence of future heart attacks and hospitalizations.

One heartening fact is that the rates of heart attacks and deaths from STEMI—the more dangerous type of heart attack—have been decreasing for years. Thanks to increased awareness, people at high risk are more likely to seek attention and receive early treatment, which helps prevent deadly cardiac events.

EARLY VS. DELAYED INVASIVE TREATMENT

In some cases of ACS, your doctor may recommend invasive treatment within the first 24 hours of your arrival at the hospital. If you're diagnosed with STEMI, a potentially dangerous type of heart attack, you will usually be referred for angiography and invasive treatment within 24 hours of the onset of your symptoms. People diagnosed with unstable angina or NSTEMI, a type of heart attack that isn't as dangerous as STEMI, and who continue to have chest pain despite the administration of medications, may also be candidates for early intervention. Similarly, people who experience some form of cardiac electrical instability—low heart rate, fast heart rate, or arrhythmia—are more likely to receive early invasive treatment.

Features for High Risk of Death
In Patients with Acute Coronary Syndrome (ACS)

⚠ Worsening chest pain over 48 hours after onset

⚠ Chest pain lasting longer than 20 minutes

⚠ Certain high-risk changes on EKG

⚠ Elevated cardiac biomarkers such as troponins

⚠ Clinical findings of acute congestive heart failure, low blood pressure, very slow or faint heart rate

⚠ Patient over age 75

For a variety of reasons, your doctor may delay invasive treatment until 24 hours have passed since your arrival at the hospital. For example, if your cardiac biomarkers are normal and you have a low risk of heart attack, your doctor will likely wait at least 24 hours before considering invasive procedures. Likewise, if you have life-threatening cancer, respiratory failure, diabetes, poor kidney function, metabolic infections, or active bleeding, the risk of intervention may outweigh the benefits.

Evaluation for Chest Pain/ACS

Immediate Initial Assessment
- Physical exam
- Check vital signs
- EKG within 10 minutes of arrival
- Take blood to test cardiac biomarkers

Immediate General Treatment
- IV access
- Start oxygen supplement if below 94%
- Activate cardiac cath lab
- Pain control with Morphine

Immediate Medications
- Aspirin: 325 mg to chew
- Nitroglycern spray under the tongue
- Emergency cholesterol-lowering med
- Betablocker meds

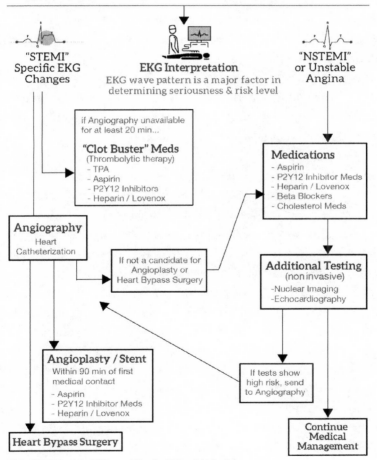

"STEMI"
Specific EKG
Changes

EKG Interpretation
EKG wave pattern is a major factor in
determining seriousness & risk level

"NSTEMI"
or Unstable
Angina

if Angiography unavailable
for at least 20 min...

"Clot Buster" Meds
(Thrombolytic therapy)
- TPA
- Aspirin
- P2Y12 Inhibitors
- Heparin / Lovenox

Medications
- Aspirin
- P2Y12 Inhibitor Meds
- Heparin / Lovenox
- Beta Blockers
- Cholesterol Meds

Angiography
Heart
Catheterization

If not a candidate for
Angioplasty or
Heart Bypass Surgery

Additional Testing
(non invasive)
-Nuclear Imaging
-Echocardiography

Angioplasty / Stent
Within 90 min of first
medical contact
- Aspirin
- P2Y12 Inhibitor Meds
- Heparin / Lovenox

If tests show
high risk, send
to Angiography

Heart Bypass Surgery

Continue
Medical
Management

*Note: STEMI stands for ST-Segment Elevation Myocardial Infarction

93

ANGIOPLASTY AND STENTS DEFINED

Angioplasty is a procedure that opens clogged arteries to improve blood flow to the heart. First performed in 1977 by Dr. Andreas Grüntzig, it revolutionized the treatment of coronary artery disease. Today, more than 600,000 people per year undergo the procedure, and it successfully opens arteries in over 90 percent of them. Compared with clot-busting medications, angioplasty is more effective at opening clogged coronary arteries and improving blood flow. In addition, angioplasty has lower risks of bleeding, repeat heart attacks, complications from heart attack, and most important, dying.

This procedure involves inserting and advancing an expandable catheter through the groin or arm. When the balloon is inflated, it pushes the plaque against the arterial walls, opening up the artery for improved blood flow. Once the artery is opened, the balloon is deflated and removed.

In most cases during angioplasty, after the balloon opens up the artery, a stent is placed to keep it open. Stents are small metal mesh tubes, introduced in the early 1990s, that widen the arteries and act as scaffolding. In some cases, scar tissue develops in the area, leading to more blockages. Stents have undergone many improvements since the first generation of bare-metal devices, however. Newer versions, known as drug-coated or drug-eluting stents, are coated with medication that helps prevent blockages from recurring. These upgraded stents also prevent the growth of scar tissue in the artery.

Patients treated with drug-coated stents also take blood thinners to prevent the formation of blood clots. In particular, physicians prescribe dual antiplatelet therapy (DAPT), a combination of aspirin and P2Y12 inhibitors, such as prasugrel, clopidogrel, or ticagrelor. In most cases, patients take an aspirin daily for the rest of their lives. The P2Y12 is usually prescribed for at least one year. Research shows that DAPT increases longevity. With the use of

DAPT, it's rare to see blockages occur in drug-coated stents.

The combination of drug-coated stents and DAPT has proven so effective that bare-metal stents are typically only used if a person can't take blood thinners. For example, if you have an increased risk of bleeding or are in need of urgent noncardiac surgery, your physician may recommend bare-metal stents.

The medical community is constantly seeking to improve the devices used to treat ACS. On the horizon is a new type of drug-coated bio-absorbable stent that dissolves over time. These stents are still in the research phase, so it is unknown when they might be available in hospitals.

Drug-Coated Stents

Name	Manufacturer	Stent Material	Drug
Xience	Abbott Vascular	Cobalt Chromium	Everolimus
Endeavor	Medtronic	Cobalt Chromium	Zotarolimus
Promus	Boston Scientific	Platinum Chromium	Everolimus
Onyx	Medtronic	Cobalt Chromium	Everolimus

ARE YOU A CANDIDATE FOR ANGIOPLASTY AND STENTING?

To determine if angioplasty and stenting is the best option for you, your doctor will look at many factors, including:

- the number of coronary arteries involved
- the location of your blockages
- the severity of your blockages
- your overall health
- how well your heart functions
- whether you have other diseases, such as diabetes or cancer
- your age

- your life expectancy
- your personal preference

In general, if your coronary artery disease involves just one or two blood vessels that can be easily reached, and you don't have diabetes, your doctor will likely recommend angioplasty and stenting. In cases of more severe coronary artery disease, or if you have diabetes, coronary artery bypass graft surgery (CABG) may also be considered.

Some doctors use the SYNTAX score to help determine which procedure to recommend. This tool helps classify the complexity of coronary artery disease based on the number and location of blockages. Other factors, such as age and kidney function, may also be weighed in determining the score. People with a higher SYNTAX score typically fare better with CABG (pronounced like the vegetable, "cabbage") while those with low to intermediate scores tend to have similar results with either procedure. You can read more about CABG in the upcoming chapter on bypass surgery.

UNDERGOING ANGIOPLASTY AND STENTING

Angioplasty is typically performed in a cath lab as part of a catheterization procedure, described in detail in Chapter 4. Although it takes place in a hospital, angioplasty is not considered major surgery and takes just 30 minutes to two hours. It is not considered painful, but you may feel some pressure as the catheter is threaded through your blood vessels, and you may experience some soreness at the insertion site following the procedure. Each procedure varies depending on the patient's particular condition and needs, but the following steps are common:

- The procedure does not require anesthesia, but you may be given a sedative to help you relax.

- An area on your groin or arm is numbed before the doctor inserts a plastic tube called a catheter into an artery.
- The doctor then threads the catheter through the blood vessel using a special monitor to see the catheter until it reaches the blocked coronary artery.
- Once the catheter is in place, a thin wire is inserted and advanced to the blockage.
- Next, a tube with an expandable balloon is passed through the catheter. In some cases, a collapsed stent is positioned over the balloon.
- The balloon is inflated, pushing the plaque against the walls of the artery to widen it.
- The balloon is deflated and removed from your body.
- If a stent is used, it remains in place to prop open the artery.
- To prevent bleeding, a healthcare professional will apply pressure to the insertion site or use a suture or plug to close the groin puncture site to prevent bleeding.
- You will need to lie on your back for several hours after the procedure to avoid bleeding.

Angioplasty & Stent Placement

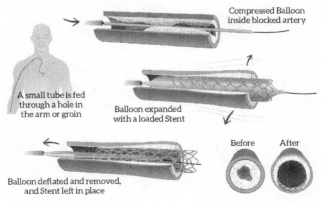

Compressed Balloon inside blocked artery

A small tube is fed through a hole in the arm or groin

Balloon expanded with a loaded Stent

Balloon deflated and removed, and Stent left in place

Before   After

When Angiograms Appear Normal

In about 7 percent of people who go to the hospital with symptoms of ACS and undergo an angiogram, there is no evidence of blockages in the coronary arteries. This occurs more often in younger patients and women. Conditions that can be present even though an angiogram looks normal include:

- Spasms of the coronary artery
- Discomfort due to cocaine abuse
- Vascular disease
- Clotting disorder
- Inflammation of the heart muscle
- Blockages in very small blood vessels that can't be seen with the naked eye
- Takotsubo cardiomyopathy

Following angioplasty, most people are discharged the same day provided their condition is stable. Some patients, however, may need to spend the night in the hospital for observation before being discharged. It's important to avoid strenuous exercise and heavy lifting for a couple days. If you notice any signs of infection—fever or redness or swelling at the insertion site—let your doctor know right away. If you experience any chest pain or if you notice bleeding at the insertion site, contact your doctor immediately or call 911.

As with all medical procedures, there are complications associated with angioplasty. The most serious complication—the sudden collapse of a widened artery—occurs in less than 5 percent of people. This rare complication usually occurs in the first few hours after the procedure when the patient is still in the hospital, so it can be treated rapidly.

INTRA-AORTIC BALLOON PUMP

Some people, like my patient Miguel, may require the insertion of an intra-aortic balloon pump (IABP), a mechanical device used to help the heart pump more blood. When an IABP is placed in the aorta, the main coronary artery that directs blood from the heart to the rest of the body, it inflates and deflates in rhythm with your heartbeat to reduce the muscle's workload. IABPs are temporary: In some cases, they remain in the body for 12 to 72 hours; in other cases, they are removed as soon as a person is stabilized. These devices are generally reserved for those who have suffered a major heart attack and also have low blood pressure.

The procedure to insert an IABP is similar to angioplasty. The balloon is inserted via a catheter injected into the groin or arm and then advanced to the aorta, where it is expanded. While the IABP is in place, you need to lie very still, which some people find uncomfortable.

A newer device similar to an IABP is the Impella heart pump, which supports and improves heart function. It is used in people who have had a severe heart attack and who also have low blood pressure or in those who are considered high risk for angioplasty procedures. The Impella heart pump can be left in a person's body for longer periods of time than a traditional IABP.

THROMBOLYTIC THERAPY

People who are not candidates for angioplasty or whose hospital doesn't offer angioplasty are often treated with thrombolytic therapy, also known as fibrinolytic therapy. Covered in Chapter 5, this clot-buster medication is often recommended in the treatment of STEMI. If these drugs do not alleviate your symptoms, you probably will be transferred to a hospital equipped for angioplasty.

CHAPTER 7

BYPASS SURGERY

Janet, 62, was working in her garden one day when she suddenly felt a sharp pain in her jaw, a tightness in her chest, and a wave of nausea. Her husband, Bill, who had suffered a heart attack a couple years earlier, recognized the signs right away and rushed her to the ER. When Janet arrived, we went to work immediately to assess her condition. In taking her medical history, we learned that she had been diagnosed with diabetes about a decade earlier. An EKG showed that Janet was having a STEMI, a dangerous type of heart attack that can damage the heart muscle, and her cardiac biomarkers were elevated. In the cath lab, we discovered that she had multiple blockages, including a severe blockage in the main coronary artery called the left main. Due to certain aspects of her coronary anatomy, Janet was recommended for coronary artery bypass graft surgery (CABG).

Janet was prepped for surgery and a few hours later, she emerged with better blood flow to her heart and minimal damage to the heart muscle. She stayed in the hospital for about a week before being discharged. At home, she faithfully took the medications I had prescribed to her. She also made it a point to do all the exercises the cardiac rehabilitation facility had recommended. And she never missed a follow-up appointment with me. The healthcare professionals at the cardiac rehab center helped keep her on track and eventually, Janet started feeling like herself again. Ten years later at age 72, Janet feels great, and her heart function is normal.

First introduced in 1967, CABG has helped millions of people restore blood flow following a heart attack. However, the number of surgeries performed has been steadily declining over the past 20 years. Thanks to improvements in angioplasty and stenting, fewer people experiencing coronary artery disease are undergoing bypass surgery. It is still considered the best option for some people, however, so it's a good idea to understand the basics of this surgery.

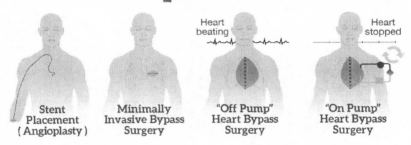

Treatment Options   Less → More Invasive

Stent Placement (Angioplasty) · Minimally Invasive Bypass Surgery · "Off Pump" Heart Bypass Surgery · "On Pump" Heart Bypass Surgery

WHAT IS BYPASS SURGERY?

Bypass surgery, or CABG, is a major surgical procedure that uses a person's own arteries and veins to bypass narrowed cardiac arteries in order to restore blood flow to the heart. A portion of one or more blood vessels is taken from another part of the body—usually the leg or chest—and then attached to arteries that are clogged, effectively creating a detour around the blockages. This improves circulation and relieves chest pain. Although CABG is a much more involved procedure than angioplasty and stenting, it is considered safe, and the two procedures have similar survival rates. People who have bypass surgery are less likely to require a repeat procedure.

Bypass Grafts

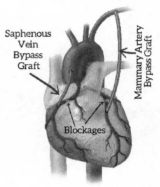

Saphenous Vein Bypass Graft

Mammary Artery Bypass Graft

Blockages

ARE YOU A CANDIDATE FOR CABG?

To determine whether bypass surgery is better for you than angioplasty and stenting, your doctor will look at the factors described earlier. In general, bypass surgery is reserved for people with:

- extensive heart disease
- multiple blockages
- blockage in the left main coronary artery
- blockages that are difficult to reach with angioplasty
- a high SYNTAX score
- poor pump function in the left ventricle
- the presence of other conditions, such as diabetes or cancer

Your doctor will take all of this into careful consideration when deciding if CABG is the best option for you.

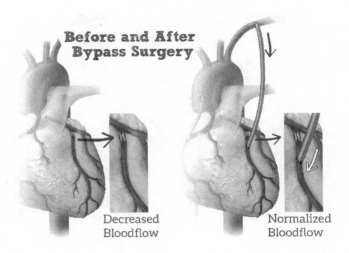

Before and After Bypass Surgery

Decreased Bloodflow

Normalized Bloodflow

UNDERGOING BYPASS SURGERY

Bypass surgery takes about three to five hours, depending on the number of blockages and where they are located. The more blockages you have and the more difficult it is to reach them, the longer the procedure will take. CABG is a major surgical procedure performed under general anesthesia, so you won't feel any pain or be awake during the operation. Your breathing, blood pressure, and oxygen levels are monitored throughout the procedure. While each procedure differs based on individual needs, the operation typically involves the following steps:

- Once you are asleep, a breathing tube is placed down your windpipe to assist your breathing during the operation, an IV line is inserted into your neck to deliver medications and to monitor your blood pressure, and a urinary catheter is inserted.

- An incision is made in the middle of your chest and a surgical saw is used to cut through your breastbone, exposing your heart.

- Your heart is cooled using a variety of techniques to reduce its need for oxygen and to prevent damage to the heart muscle.
- Portions of one or more blood vessels are harvested, usually from your leg (the saphenous vein) or chest (the internal mammary artery, or IMA). To harvest the saphenous vein, an incision is made on the inside of one or both legs. If the IMA is being used, no additional incision is necessary.
- One end of the harvested blood vessel is attached directly to the aorta, and the other end is affixed beyond the blockage, creating a detour past the blockage. In some cases, an artery from the arm (called a radial artery graft) or abdomen (called a gastroepiploic graft) may be used.
- Your surgeon ensures the grafts are functioning properly before closing your incisions.

Heart Bypass Surgery
CABG = Coronary Artery Bypass Graft

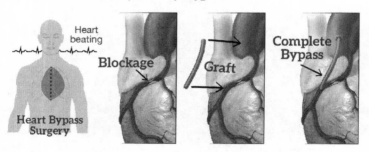

TYPES OF CABG PROCEDURES

On-pump: About 85 to 90 percent of all bypass surgeries are performed as "on-pump" procedures. This means your heart is temporarily stopped and put on a heart-lung machine, also known as a cardiopulmonary bypass. This device takes over your heart's pumping action, diverting blood away from your heart, adding oxygen to it, and delivering it to the rest of your body. It involves placing a clamp on the heart's biggest vessel, the aorta. Trained specialists called perfusion technologists oversee the heart-lung machine during the procedure. The heart-lung machine keeps your heart still, allowing your surgeon to work with greater precision on your coronary arteries. After the grafts have been placed, your heart will be taken off the heart-lung machine and given an electric shock to resume beating.

Off-pump: In some cases, your surgeon may opt not to use the heart-lung machine, which is referred to as an "off-pump" procedure. This may be recommended if you are at a high risk of complications, such as a stroke. In people with severe calcification in the aorta, there is a risk that clamping the aorta will cause clots to dislodge and travel to other parts of the body. Performing bypass surgery on a beating heart, however, is more challenging and requires a highly trained surgeon.

ADDITIONAL BYPASS SURGERY TECHNIQUES

MIDCAB: The minimally invasive direct coronary artery bypass (MIDCAB) involves an alternative incision site. Rather than making an incision in the center of the chest, a surgeon makes a smaller incision through the chest directly over your heart. There is no need to cut through the breastbone or to open the ribcage with MIDCAB. The surgeon can access the coronary arteries in between the ribs.

Most of these procedures are performed on a beating heart, so they do not require you to be on a heart-lung machine. For this reason, MIDCAB is considered an off-pump procedure. Typically, MIDCAB is used only in people who have just one or two clogged arteries that can be bypassed using the internal mammary artery.

MIDCAB typically results in fewer complications and requires fewer recovery days in the hospital.

Surgery for Bypasses:
Traditional vs Minimally Invasive

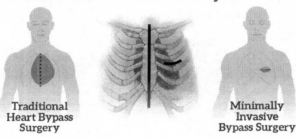

Traditional Heart Bypass Surgery	Minimally Invasive Bypass Surgery
The breastbone and rib cage are cut open to reach the heart. Graft veins are placed on the heart to bypass any blockages.	MIDCAB A small hole is cut between ribs to reach the heart. A graft vein is placed on the heart to bypass a blockage.

Hybrid: In some cases, your doctor may recommend a hybrid approach that involves CABG and the placement of stents during angioplasty. This combination approach is performed in one of two ways.

- **Staged procedure:** With a staged procedure, stenting and bypass surgery are scheduled on separate occasions.
- **Combination procedure:** With a combination procedure, angioplasty, stent placement, and bypass surgery are performed at the same time. For this approach, an interventional cardiologist and a cardiothoracic surgeon work in tandem. Most often, the surgeon uses the MIDCAB procedure to place a graft in the heart's main artery, the left anterior descending artery. The cardiologist then follows up with angioplasty and stenting to open up any other clogged arteries.

The "Hybrid" Approach for Multiple Blockages

Decision for each blockage ...
Clear it or bypass it?

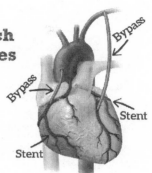

Bypass

Bypass

Stent

Stent

RECOVERING FROM BYPASS SURGERY

Following bypass surgery, you are sent to the intensive care unit (ICU) for observation. When the anesthesia wears off and you wake up and are breathing on your own, the breathing tube is removed. You may have a sore throat due to the breathing tube, but it usually goes away within a few days. Once you can stand up and urinate on your own, the urinary catheter is removed. The IV line in your neck remains for a few days to administer fluids and medications and to continuously monitor your blood pressure. While in the ICU, you are monitored closely for pain, and medications are administered accordingly to minimize any discomfort.

After a few days, you will likely be transferred to an intermediate care unit, where you will continue to be monitored for pain and any complications. The amount of time you spend in the hospital depends on which type of bypass surgery procedure you have and whether you experience any complications.

COMPLICATIONS OF BYPASS SURGERY

As with any surgery, there are risks associated with CABG. In general, the risk of complications is low, but it also depends on your individual condition and your overall health prior to the operation. Possible complications include the following:

- *Constipation:* Taking pain medication can cause constipation. This usually resolves when you stop taking the pain relief medication. In the meantime, you may want to use a laxative or stool softener.
- *Leg swelling:* Temporary swelling of the legs may occur following bypass surgery. You may need to raise the foot of your hospital bed while you are lying down or put pillows underneath your feet to elevate them. You may also be instructed to wear support hose to prevent swelling.
- *Damage to heart muscle:* About 2 to 4 percent of bypass surgery patients experience damage to the heart muscle during bypass surgery. This can be detected using EKG and ultrasound. In most cases, the damage is minor and easily treated while you are in the hospital. In rare cases when there is more damage, you may need a temporary intra-aortic balloon pump (IABP) or left ventricle assist device (LVAD) while the heart muscle heals.
- *Arrythmia:* Irregular heart rhythms can occur as a complication of bypass surgery. Atrial fibrillation, in which the heart beats chaotically, is the most common type of arrhythmia seen in bypass surgery patients. About 40 percent of people who develop arrhythmia after CABG have atrial fibrillation. This can be controlled with medication. More serious types of arrhythmia that may occur include ventricular tachycardia, ventricular fibrillation, and bradycardia. Post-surgical arrhythmias can usually be controlled with medication and do not require a pacemaker.

- *Bleeding:* About 30 percent of people who undergo bypass surgery require a blood transfusion.
- *Fluid around the lungs:* Up to 10 percent of bypass surgery patients will accumulate fluid around the lungs, which is called pleural effusion. If you experience a buildup of fluid, your doctor may prescribe medications called diuretics. In some cases, you may require a procedure called thoracentesis, which involves placing a needle through the back to drain the fluid around the lungs.
- *Stroke:* About 2 to 4 percent of patients experience a stroke after undergoing bypass surgery.
- *Confusion and memory changes:* Following bypass surgery, patients often experience temporary changes in cognitive thinking and memory. This is usually temporary. If your cognitive skills don't improve, talk to your doctor.
- *Anxiety and depression:* It is not uncommon for people who have had bypass surgery to sink into a state of depression or to experience heightened anxiety. Women are 40 percent more likely than men to experience these psychological effects. Be sure to let your doctor know about any changes in your mental state.
- *Infection:* About 1 percent of patients get an infection at the incision site. This is more common in people who are obese or who have diabetes and in women who have breast cancer. Antibiotics are used to heal the infection.
- *Leg wounds:* About 5 percent of people who have had veins harvested from their legs develop some form of wound. This can be treated with antibiotics and wound care.
- *Decrease in kidney function:* Some people may see their kidney function deteriorate, but this is usually temporary.
- *Phrenic nerve damage:* Damage to the phrenic nerve, which controls your diaphragm, occurs in about 1 percent of

bypass surgery patients. This can affect your breathing and requires treatment.

- *Damage to the intercostal nerves:* Rarely, the intercostal nerves, which are part of the somatic nervous system, can be damaged. This may lead to numbness and pain in the chest area.

- *Aortic dissection:* In very rare cases, the aorta may tear as a result of bypass surgery. This catastrophic event can be fatal. Elderly people with high blood pressure are at the highest risk of this complication.

- *Thrombocytopenia:* In some people who have bypass surgery, platelet levels may decrease to abnormally low levels. This increases the risk of bleeding. Medical professionals believe this may be due to the use of the blood thinner heparin. If this occurs, you will be closely monitored and treated with medication.

RECOVERING AT HOME

Once you are discharged from the hospital and return home, you will begin to resume your life, with some important changes.

- *Medications:* You will likely have a number of new medications to take. To ensure your swift recovery, be sure to take all medications as prescribed by your doctor.

- *Wound care:* After your stitches or staples have been removed—usually within a week or so of your surgery— you will be advised how to clean and care for the incision sites.

- *Resuming sexual activity:* Most people can safely resume sexual activity about two weeks after a heart attack; however, sexual problems occur in more than 50 percent of patients. Some people fear that sexual activity may lead to another heart attack. New medications may affect sexual performance. Anxiety and depression may impact libido. In men, erectile dysfunction may occur. All of these issues can be treated with counseling and medications.

- *Driving:* Most people can begin driving about four to six weeks after surgery.
- *Working:* If you have a desk job, you can probably return to work in about four weeks. If your job involves physical labor, you'll need to wait longer.
- *Walking:* Although you should avoid strenuous exercise and heavy lifting at first, you will be encouraged to walk. Going for a walk is one of the best ways to regain your strength.

CARDIAC REHABILITATION PROGRAM

Your doctor will also recommend that you participate in cardiac rehabilitation, which is a supervised exercise program. Cardiac rehab usually takes place in an outpatient facility, but some elderly patients may do a hospital-based exercise program. Cardiac rehab is covered by most health insurance plans and offers many benefits, including:

- improves wound healing
- lowers heart rate
- reduces risk of complications
- improves exercise ability
- decreases stress, anxiety, and depression
- helps control other risk factors, including diabetes, high blood pressure, and high cholesterol
- Typically, you will go to cardiac rehab a few times per week, and your workout will consist of:
  - five to 10 minutes of warm-up
  - 15 to 20 minutes of exercise

- five minutes of cool-down

Trained clinicians will work with you based on your fitness level prior to bypass surgery. The intensity of your workout will also depend on your heart rate and how well your heart functions. If your heart function is compromised, you'll start with a gentler workout. The better your heart functions, the more intense your workout. As your heart function and performance improve, you will progress to the next level. You will also receive instructions on how to perform certain exercises so you can do them at home on the days you don't go to the rehab facility.

The cardiac rehab clinicians assist with far more than just physical exercise. They can help you quit smoking, offer support and resources for anxiety and depression, and much more.

CHAPTER 8

TREATING COMPLICATIONS OF A HEART ATTACK

L amar, a retired attorney, suffered a heart attack at age 71 due to a blocked right coronary artery. He underwent angioplasty, and stents were placed in his coronary artery. The procedure went smoothly, and Lamar left the hospital with some new medications and instructions for diet and exercise. His wife, Sherelle, was a nurse, so she made sure Lamar took his medication, ate right, and kept up with his workouts. Lamar did everything right, so he was shocked when he ended up with a complication. "I did everything you told me to do," he said during one of his follow-up appointments. "So why did this happen to me?"

I explained to him that even though he was a model patient, complications can still occur. In his case, his heart began beating irregularly, something that isn't uncommon among heart attack survivors. I diagnosed Lamar with atrial fibrillation, a condition which can lead to other complications, such as blood clots, and needs to be treated. Lamar began taking antiarrhythmic drugs, which helped restore a more rhythmic heartbeat.

Surviving a heart attack is a great feeling. Like Lamar, you may think that once the immediate danger is past, you're in the clear.

But there is still a possibility that you might experience compli-cations. These additional issues can range from mild setbacks to life-threatening conditions. In the hours, weeks, and months after a heart attack, your condition will be monitored closely so you can receive early treatment in the event you experience any of the fol-lowing complications. Be sure to report any changes in your physi-cal or mental health to your doctor right away.

RHYTHM DISORDERS

One of the more common complications from a heart attack is arrhythmia, which means your heart beats too fast (tachycardia), too slow (bradycardia), or in an irregular tempo (atrial fibrillation). A normal heart beats 60 to 100 times per minute when you are at rest. Arrhythmia can develop as a consequence of damage to the heart muscle, and this damage can disrupt the electrical signals that regulate your heartbeat. The risk of rhythm problems is high-est in the first 12 to 24 hours following a heart attack and remains for the first six months.

When your heartbeat is out of rhythm, it may be a benign nui-sance or a life-threatening problem. Arrhythmia can result from damaged heart muscle or electrolyte imbalances and abnormal levels of magnesium. In extreme cases, it may require treat-ment with shocks, medication, or a pacemaker. For this reason, it's imperative to tell your doctor if you notice any symptoms of arrhythmia.

- *Tachycardia:* When your heart beats too fast—more than 100 beats per minute—it can cause a variety of symptoms, includ-ing palpitations (the feeling that your heart is racing out of control), high pulse rate, fainting, lightheadedness, dizziness, fatigue, and chest pain. Complications of tachycardia include blood clots, heart failure, and sudden cardiac death.

- *Bradycardia:* If your heartbeat slows to fewer than 60 beats per minute, you may experience symptoms such as fainting, fatigue, lightheadedness, dizziness, shortness of breath, chest pain, confusion, memory problems, and exhaustion with physical exertion. Surprisingly, many symptoms of a slow heartbeat and a fast heartbeat are the same. Complications of bradycardia include fainting spells, heart failure, and sudden cardiac death.

- *Atrial fibrillation:* When the heart beats in an irregular, chaotic fashion, it can produce symptoms such as palpitations, shortness of breath, and weakness. Seen in 10 to 20 percent of people who have a heart attack, atrial fibrillation may last for just a few seconds or may not go away without treatment. Complications of atrial fibrillation include blood clots, stroke, and heart failure.

PERICARDITIS

After a heart attack, the two layers of tissue that surround the heart—the pericardium—may become inflamed. This condition, called pericarditis, can cause the two layers to rub against each other or against the heart, resulting in chest pain. It occurs in about 10 to 12 percent of people who have a heart attack. Early treatment with angioplasty reduces the incidence of pericarditis.

The onset of this complication usually happens one to four days after a heart attack. Symptoms include a low-grade fever, specific sounds that can be heard with a stethoscope, and chest pain. An EKG will show certain changes indicating pericarditis. If your doctor suspects this complication, you may be required to undergo an ultrasound to ensure there is no fluid around the heart. Pericarditis is usually treated with medication, such as anti-inflammatory drugs.

Dressler's syndrome: A type of pericarditis, Dressler's syndrome may occur two to five weeks after a heart attack. When cardiac tissue is injured due to a heart attack, the body's natural immune response system goes into action to repair the damage. In some cases, this can lead to inflammation, which can cause symptoms of fever and chest pain. In severe cases, this condition is treated with steroids and anti-inflammatory medication. Your chances of developing Dressler's syndrome are reduced if you receive early treatment with clot-busting medication.

BLOOD CLOT DISORDERS
A blood clot that clogs a coronary artery can dislodge and travel through the blood vessel to other bodily organs. If a blood clot goes to the brain, it can cause a stroke. A clot that heads to the legs is called a peripheral embolism. These conditions can be life threatening and need immediate medical attention.

RUPTURE OF THE HEART WALL
When the heart muscle is damaged due to a lack of blood flow, it can lead to a rupture in the heart wall. The rupture allows blood to leak into the surrounding sac, called the pericardium, and can be fatal. The incidence of this catastrophic complication, seen in less than 1 percent of people who suffer a heart attack, is declining thanks to medications and invasive techniques that quickly open clogged arteries and, in turn, reduce the incidence of heart attacks. Symptoms of a rupture include chest pain, nausea, and low blood pressure. Doctors typically use ultrasound to make a diagnosis. When the heart wall tears, it requires emergency surgery during which a needle is inserted into the cavity surrounding the heart to relieve pressure.

HEART MUSCLE DYSFUNCTION
In some cases, a heart attack may cause such extensive damage to the heart muscle that it can no longer function adequately as a

pump. This can result in blood and fluid accumulating in the lungs, impacting the ability to breathe, causing blood pressure to plummet to dangerously low levels, and reducing oxygen saturation levels. People who suffer from this type of dysfunction may be treated with medications, an IABP, or bypass surgery.

LEFT VENTRICLE ANEURYSM

After a heart attack, poor circulation can change the texture of the heart muscle, thinning its tissues. In rare cases, this may lead to a small swelling in the left ventricle called an aneurysm. If left untreated, the aneurysm can burst. It's important to identify and treat any swelling in the left ventricle early to avoid a tear. Specific changes on an EKG give doctors a clue that there may be an aneurysm, and a follow-up ultrasound can confirm it. People who develop this condition may need to undergo surgery to remove the aneurysm from the ventricle.

RIGHT VENTRICULAR FAILURE

The right ventricle's job is to pump blood from the heart to the lungs. After a heart attack that affects the right ventricle, however, it may lose some of its pumping ability. This can lead to a buildup of fluid in the body, causing swelling in the ankles, legs, and abdomen. An ultrasound can detect this condition, which may be treated with IV fluids and angioplasty to treat any blockages.

LEAKY HEART VALVE

Following a heart attack, it's possible to develop a leaky heart valve, which cardiologists refer to as acute mitral regurgitation. The mitral valve normally allows blood to pass from the left atrium to the left ventricle. In a healthy heart, the blood flows only in this direction. Depending on damage from a heart attack, however, blood may also flow backward, causing the left atrium to become overloaded with blood. This increases pressure and can lead to symptoms including palpitations, chest pain, shortness of breath, fatigue, and swollen ankles and feet. Diagnosed using ultrasound, a leaky valve may require emergency surgery to repair it.

HOLE IN THE HEART (VENTRICULAR SEPTAL DEFECT)

The ventricular septum is a membrane that separates the right and left ventricles of the heart. This wall helps keep blood flowing in a one-way direction through the heart's four chambers. In rare cases, however, a heart attack can cause a thinning of the septum's tissue, wearing it down until a hole develops. This complication is most commonly seen in the elderly, women, people experiencing a first heart attack, and those with very high blood pressure.

Usually seen within the first seven days of a heart attack, this hole, called a ventricular septal defect, allows oxygenated and unoxygenated blood to comingle in the two chambers. This makes you extremely short of breath and may lead to respiratory failure and heart failure. This potentially fatal condition requires surgery to close the hole.

DEPRESSION

After a heart attack, it's normal to experience a range of emotions, including sadness, fear, and anger. In most people, these feelings resolve over time. In up to 33 percent of people, however, depression sets in. There is also an increased risk of suicide following a heart attack. If you have experienced a heart attack, be conscious of your mental state and talk to your doctor if you are no longer finding joy in your life or if you are having suicidal thoughts. Medication and other treatment options can help you regain a more positive outlook.

PART III

LIVING WITH CORONARY HEART

DISEASE

*"Tend to your vital heart, and all that you worry
about will be solved."*
— Rumi

CHAPTER 9

EAT HEART-HEALTHY FOODS

After experiencing a heart attack or receiving a diagnosis of coronary heart disease (CHD), my patients inevitably ask me what they should be eating to prevent any future coronary events. And in many cases, my patients' spouses and adult children ask for dietary advice on how to prevent CHD. Research shows that eating a heart-healthy diet can play an important role in lowering cholesterol levels, improving arterial function, and reducing the risk of heart attack. But finding the right diet can be tricky.

Many of my patients and their families have searched for a heart-healthy eating plan only to be left more confused than when they started. It's no surprise. Turn on the TV, pick up a magazine, or do a quick internet search, and you're likely to be bombarded with conflicting messages from diet gurus, nutrition bloggers, and medical experts promising better health. With such a glut of information, it's difficult to figure out what's best. After more than two decades as a cardiologist, I've discovered that there isn't a one-size-fits-all solution. Each heart patient is different.

Take Jerry, for example. He suffered a heart attack at age 62 and underwent coronary bypass graft surgery. Jerry tipped the scales at over 300 pounds, and his cholesterol and triglyceride levels were through the roof. In follow-up appointments with me, he filled me in on his typical eating habits—steak and eggs for breakfast, steak sandwich for lunch, and steak and potatoes for dinner. I informed Jerry that being obese was increasing his risk of another coronary event, and his steak habit wasn't helping him. Together, we came up with a plan to swap out his daily steaks in favor of fish, poultry, and legumes. Considering how high Jerry's cholesterol levels were, I also prescribed statins.

Within six months, Jerry had lost over 50 pounds and his lipid levels had dropped into the normal range. Now several years later, Jerry is down to 180 pounds, his cholesterol and triglycerides remain at a healthy level, and his other diagnostic tests show no signs of heart disease. He still enjoys an occasional steak, but he's grown to love more variety in his meals.

My patient Sarah, who required angioplasty and stenting at age 58, had a different story. She thought she was following a heart-healthy diet because she never ate red meat and avoided most saturated fats. Plus, she watched her calories and still weighed the same as she had in college. What wasn't working in her favor was that despite having high blood pressure, she was filling up on high-sodium soups, crackers, and baked goods, as well as sugary treats and sodas—all of which can contribute to heart disease.

I encouraged Sarah to limit her sodium intake, trade in sugary desserts for low-fat yogurt and fruit, and increase her consumption of fiber-rich whole grains. With time, Sarah's blood pressure improved so much she was able to stop taking medication. By getting her blood pressure under control, Sarah reduced her risk of heart attack and stroke.

With Jerry and Sarah, I didn't recommend or endorse one particular regimented diet plan. Instead, I shared general heart-healthy dietary guidelines that have the most evidence-based science to back them up. In general, I try to keep it simple for my patients.

In this chapter, I'll reveal the basic eating habits shown to have the most benefit for improving lipid profiles and preventing, slowing, or reversing CHD. From these core guidelines, you can tailor a plan to fit your specific needs. And don't worry. Eating a heart-healthy diet doesn't mean you have to ditch all your favorite foods. With some easy swaps, you can fill your body with nutrient-rich fare that tastes great and keeps you feeling great.

DIETARY GUIDELINES
from the American Heart Association

Caloric intake:
- Fat should be <30% of total calories
- Saturated fat should be <10% of total calories
- Polyunsaturated fat consumption should be <300 mg/day
- Carbohydrates (especially complex type) should constitute 1/2 of calories in diet
- Protein should constitute the remainder
- Calories should be sufficient to maintain an optimal body weight

Sodium intake: < 2400 mg / day

Alcohol intake: ≤ 60g (2 oz) / day

LIMIT FATS

Decades of clinical research have shown that reducing dietary fat intake is beneficial for people with CHD. The American Heart Association (AHA) recommends limiting fat intake to no more than 30 percent of your total daily calories. Be aware, not all fat is the same. It's a good idea to understand the different types of fat so you know which ones are harmful to heart health and which ones offer some protection. With this knowledge, you can limit or eliminate your intake of bad fats and emphasize good fats in your meals.

Saturated Fats

Saturated fats are considered "bad fats" because they increase cholesterol levels, particularly LDL, which is the bad type of cholesterol. Saturated fats are derived primarily from animal sources, such meat and dairy. In addition, certain plant-based oils—

Foods High in Saturated Fats

- Fatty beef
- Poultry (with skin)
- Lamb
- Pork
- Butter
- Cheese
- Whole milk
- Ice cream
- Coconut oil
- Palm oil
- Palm kernel oil

such as palm oil, palm kernel oil, and coconut oil—are sources of saturated fats. It's easy to identify saturated fats: They are solid at room temperature.

As a rule of thumb, I advise limiting your intake of saturated fats. The AHA and the American College of Cardiology (ACC) suggest lowering your saturated fat intake to about 5 to 6 percent of your total daily calories. In people with elevated LDL levels, this has been shown to reduce the incidence of coronary events, such as heart attack or acute coronary syndrome (ACS), and improve overall heart health.

Keep in mind the average daily intake of saturated fats is about 10 to 12 percent of total calories, so the AHA and ACC are recommending to cut that amount in half. For example, let's say you eat 2,000 calories per day. In this case, you should aim for no more than 100 to 120 calories of saturated fat per day.

Maximum Daily Saturated Fat Calories Allowed

Total Daily Calories	Maximum Saturated Fat Calories Allowed
2,000	100-120
1,800	90-108
1,500	75-90

The maximum saturated fat calories allowed are based on 5 to 6 percent of total daily calories.

How do you calculate how many saturated fat calories are in a food item? It's easy. One gram of fat equals 9 calories. Simply take the number of saturated fat grams (it's listed on food labels) and multiply by 9 to arrive at the number of saturated fat calories. For example, if one serving of a particular food has 5 grams of saturated fat, multiply that number by 9. The result is 45 calories.

How to Calculate Saturated Fat Calories

- 1 gram of saturated fat = 9 calories

- Multiply grams of saturated fat by 9

- Number of grams x 9 = calories

Considering that many popular diet gurus these days promote coconut oil as a heart-healthy food, you may be wondering why I don't recommend it. Coconut oil is rich in saturated fat, which, according to decades of research, raises LDL and the risk of CHD. Despite claims to the contrary found on the internet, there is no good scientific evidence that coconut oil reduces CHD.

Trans Fats

Trans fats raise "lousy" LDL while decreasing HDL, the "happy" or protective type of cholesterol. Consuming foods made with trans fats increases your risk of CHD, as well as stroke and Type 2 diabetes. Trace amounts of natural trans fats are found in some animal and dairy products, but these don't have a significant effect on cholesterol levels. Artificial trans fats, however, are far more prevalent in the average American diet and are a major contributor to abnormal cholesterol levels.

Trans fats are created artificially through a process that adds hydrogen to liquid vegetable oils to render them more solid. Food manufacturers use trans fats for a variety of reasons. In addition to being inexpensive to create, they lengthen a product's shelf life, enhance flavor, and improve texture. Head down the aisles of any

Common Foods with Trans Fats

- Cakes
- Cupcakes
- Cookies
- Crackers
- Doughnuts
- French fries
- Biscuits
- Microwave popcorn
- Pies
- Frozen pizza
- Stick margarine

grocery store, and you'll find the shelves packed with products that include trans fats. These bad fats are commonly found in store-bought cakes, cookies, crackers, biscuits, and stick margarine. Trans fats are also popular at some restaurants and fast food outlets that deep-fry foods, such as doughnuts and french fries. Due to public outcry about the harmful effects of trans fats, some manufacturers and restaurants are removing them from their product lines and menu offerings.

Because trans fats are so detrimental to a person's cholesterol profile and overall heart health, you should eliminate them as much as possible from your diet. To do so, you need to become a savvy nutrition label reader. Check the food labels of every product you buy, and go online to look up the nutrition information for your favorite restaurants.

Monounsaturated and Polyunsaturated Fats

Monounsaturated fats (MUFAs) and polyunsaturated fats (PUFAs) are considered "good" fats that have a beneficial effect on heart health. Clinical trials show that these fats reduce LDL and triglyceride levels, raise HDL, and lower the risk of coronary events by about 30 percent. This is similar to what is achieved by statin therapy alone. For this reason, I recommend adding these beneficial fats to your diet, especially if you've been diagnosed with CHD or had a heart attack.

Although MUFAs and PUFAs are considered good fats, they are still fats and should be used in moderation. Like other fats, they have 9 calories per gram. Compared with saturated fats, which are solid at room temperature, MUFAs and PUFAs are liquid at room temperature.

MUFAs and PUFAs are found primarily in vegetable oils, certain types of fish, nuts, and seeds. These foods are rich in essential fatty acids, including omega-3, omega-6, and alpha-linolenic acid (ALA). Your body requires these essential fats for optimal functioning, but it can't produce them naturally. The only way to get them is to absorb them from your food.

Fatty fish that are high in omega-3 fatty acids include salmon, trout, tuna, mackerel, sardines, and herring. Flaxseeds and walnuts also provide a good dose of beneficial omega-3 fatty acids. Among vegetable oils, olive oil is particularly high in MUFAs and omega-3 fatty acids.

Other vegetable oils are higher in omega-6 fatty acids and ALA. Soybean and corn oils are rich in omega-6 fatty acids. Canola and soybean oils are good sources of ALA, providing about 10 percent and 7 percent of this essential fatty acid, respectively. Sunflower oil is rich in both MUFAs and PUFAs and has been shown to reduce LDL but appears to have no effect on HDL, according to research.

Olive oil, and in particular extra-virgin olive oil (EVOO), is the principal source of fat in the Mediterranean diet and has been evaluated in numerous studies. The results are clear: EVOO reduces LDL and raises HDL. This effect is due in part to polyphenols found in the oil. Polyphenols are antioxidants that fight the aging process and help prevent diseases, such as CHD, cancer, diabetes, and high blood pressure. In terms of heart health, polyphenols don't just help raise HDL levels, but they also increase the size of HDL lipoproteins and improve their stability. Studies have shown that consuming a Mediterranean diet, which is rich in EVOO, significantly reduces incidence of heart attack and stroke and lowers the death rate from these events.

Common Sources of MUFAs and/or PUFAs

- Canola oil
- Corn oil
- Flaxseeds
- Herring
- Mackerel
- Olive oil
- Peanut oil
- Safflower oil
- Salmon
- Sardines
- Sesame oil
- Soybean oil
- Sunflower oil
- Trout
- Tuna
- Walnuts

To obtain adequate amounts of good fats, eat fatty fish at least twice a week, have a few nuts a couples times a week, and use small amounts of these vegetable oils in your meals. If you aren't getting enough healthy fats, consider adding omega-3 fatty acid supplements to your diet. (See more on supplements later in this chapter.)

LIMIT THE SWEET STUFF

Did you know that American adults gobble up an average of 22 teaspoons of added sugars every day? That's more than 8,000 teaspoons, or about 165 cups, per year. Eating too many added sugars may lead to high cholesterol, diabetes, obesity, and high blood sugar—all of which contribute to CHD. Even worse, new research shows that the more added sugars you consume, the greater your risk of dying from CHD. Be aware that *added* sugars are the real culprit here. Natural sugars found in whole fruits are considered beneficial for people with CHD.

Added sugars are prevalent in our food supply. It's no surprise that they're abundant in sweet treats like candy, cake, and ice cream. But these sneaky sugars also show up in some unexpected foods like salad dressings, barbecue sauce, and whole-grain bread.

Cutting back on added sugars is a key component of a heart-healthy diet. The AHA recommends limiting daily consumption of added sugars to no more than 6 teaspoons (about 100 calories) for women and 9 teaspoons (150 calories) for men. To reduce your intake of added sugars, check food labels to root out hidden sugars. Look for labels that say "no added sugars" or "unsweetened."

If you absolutely must indulge your sweet tooth, try nibbling on some dark chocolate. Studies show that it may be beneficial for heart health when eaten in moderation. The key word here is "moderation." A couple squares from a chocolate bar, or up to 1 ounce, is enough to gain the benefits without overdoing it.

REDUCE SODIUM INTAKE

If you're one of those people who sprinkle salt on their food before even tasting it, it may come as no surprise that you might be getting too much sodium in your diet. But did you know that even if you never use the salt shaker, you could still be consuming too much sodium? The majority of the sodium Americans eat doesn't come from the salt shaker. It comes from processed, canned, frozen, packaged, and restaurant foods.

What exactly is sodium, and is it the same as table salt? Many people use

Foods and Beverages with Added Sugars

- Sodas
- Fruit drinks
- Sports drinks
- Alcohol mixers
- Sweetened teas
- Sugary coffee drinks
- Vitamin and "health" waters
- Milk alternatives
- Candy
- Chocolate
- Bread
- Cake
- Cinnamon rolls
- Cookies
- Doughnuts
- Granola bars
- Muffins
- Ice cream
- Frozen yogurt
- Flavored yogurt
- Salad dressing
- Barbecue sauce
- Marinara sauce
- Peanut butter

Top 10 Foods Contributing to Sodium Consumption

Forty percent of the sodium consumed in the U.S. comes from the following 10 foods:

- Breads and rolls
- Cold cuts/cured meats
- Pizza
- Poultry (fresh and processed)
- Soups
- Sandwiches (such as cheeseburgers)
- Cheese
- Pasta dishes (such as spaghetti with meat sauce)
- Meat-mixed dishes (such as meatloaf with tomato sauce)
- Snacks (such as pretzels and potato chips)

Source: CDC, Vital Signs: Foods Contributing the Most to Sodium Consumption—United States 2007-2008

the terms "salt" and "sodium" interchangeably, but table salt is actually a blend of sodium and chloride, which are both minerals. Sodium is critical to our survival. It plays an essential role in keeping nerves and muscles functioning properly and helps balance fluids in the body. When too much sodium enters the bloodstream, blood vessels absorb and retain additional water to dilute the sodium. This increases the amount of blood in your vessels, which raises blood pressure and makes your heart work harder. As you've seen in this book, elevated blood pressure is a contributing risk factor of CHD.

Reducing the amount of sodium in your diet can be helpful in lowering your risk of high blood pressure, CHD, and stroke. In general, it's recommended that you skip the salt shaker and lower your sodium intake to no more than 2,400mg per day. Note that just 1 teaspoon of table salt has about 2,300mg of sodium. If you have high blood pressure, you should reduce your intake to less than 1,500mg of sodium per day. Because sodium is so prevalent in our food supply, check nutrition labels carefully and look for items that say "low salt" or "low sodium."

Specific Food Items

Specific Food Items	Recommendation
Sugar-sweetened beverages	Avoid
Processed or organ-based meats	Avoid
Fried foods	Avoid
Foods with added fats	Avoid
Eggs	Avoid
Dietary cholesterol	Limit
Coconut oil, Palm oil	Avoid
Antioxidant supplements	Avoid
Canola oil, Sunflower oil, Olive oil	In moderation
Nuts	In moderation
Antioxidant-rich fruits and vegetables	Frequent
Green leafy vegetables	Frequent
Protein from plant sources	Frequent
Gluten-containing foods	Avoid if sensitive or allergic

Freeman, A.M. et al. J am Coll Cardiol. 2017;69(9):1172-87

ADD FRUITS AND VEGETABLES

Fruits and vegetables are an important part of a heart-healthy diet. High in vitamins, minerals, and other important nutrients, these foods are considered disease fighters that may reduce the risk of CHD, cancer, diabetes, and other conditions. In addition, fruits and veggies are high in fiber and low in fat and calories, which means you can fill up on them guilt-free. In fact, the AHA recommends consuming about 4½ cups each of fruits and veggies per day. Take note that avocados, olives, and coconuts have a higher fat content and should be consumed in moderation.

For optimal health, I typically recommend eating fruits and vegetables from a rainbow of colors. Think green (broccoli, grapes, spinach), red (apples, beets, strawberries), yellow/orange (oranges, carrots, yams), blue/purple (blueberries, eggplant, plums), and white/tan (bananas, cauliflower, mushrooms).

GO FOR WHOLE GRAINS

To eat smart for your heart, be sure to consume whole grains, such as oats, whole wheat, brown rice, and quinoa. Grains are derived from the plant seeds. Like their name implies, whole grains contain the entire seed, which consists of the bran, germ, and endosperm. Whole grains are packed with nutrients, including B vitamins, iron, magnesium, and selenium. They are also a good source of fiber, which keeps you feeling full and helps lower cholesterol levels.

By contrast, refined grains—found in foods like white bread, cakes, cookies, and pizza crust—have been stripped of the bran and germ, giving them a finer texture. Food manufacturers may artificially enrich refined grains with vitamins, but they don't replace the fiber content. For this reason, it is not advisable to consume refined grains.

In whole grains, there are two types of dietary fiber: soluble and insoluble. Both play a role in heart health.

Soluble fiber: In the body, soluble fiber absorbs water and turns into a gel-like substance. This sticky goo attaches to dietary cholesterol in your digestive tract and transports it out of the body, effectively decreasing the amount that is absorbed into the bloodstream. Because of this, soluble fibers reduce cholesterol levels, particularly LDL. When you eat foods with soluble fiber, such as oats, be sure to drink plenty of water to keep your digestive system moving smoothly.

Insoluble fiber: Insoluble fibers, found in grains like brown rice and whole wheat, don't dissolve in water. They can't be digested and add bulk to your stool to help keep you regular. Evidence shows that consuming insoluble fiber reduces the risk of CHD and slows its progression in people at high risk.

To make sure you are choosing healthy whole grains, read food labels carefully. The first ingredient should include the word "whole," as in "whole wheat" or "whole oats." Check the number of grams of dietary fiber as well—more is better. Whole grains include higher amounts of dietary fiber compared with refined fiber. You can also look for the "Whole Grain" stamp from the Whole Grains Council, which certifies a food as 100 percent whole grain.

Examples of Whole Grains

- Barley
- Buckwheat
- Bulghur
- Corn
- Millet
- Oats/oatmeal
- Popcorn
- Quinoa
- Rice (brown, wild)
- Rye
- Whole wheat

STICK TO LEAN PROTEINS

Most Americans eat a very protein-rich diet. Proteins provide key nutrients, such as vitamin D, iron, and zinc. The problem is that much of our protein comes in the shape of meats laden with saturated fats, which elevate LDL levels. One of the keys to heart-healthy eating is to choose proteins that are low in these fats. Fortunately, there are many delicious sources of lean proteins, including fish, white-meat chicken and turkey (without skin), low-fat or nonfat dairy, legumes, and soy products (tofu and tempeh).

What about eggs? For years, cardiologists have warned patients to steer clear of eggs and especially their sunny yolks. That's because eggs, although rich in protein, are high in cholesterol. One large egg provides about 6 grams of protein but contains about 180g of cholesterol. For comparison purposes, 4 ounces of chicken breast (skin and fat removed) offers about 35g of protein but only about 90g of cholesterol.

A diet high in egg consumption is associated with a greater risk of CHD, especially in people with diabetes. For this reason, I typically recommend limiting your intake to no more than one egg per day.

Similarly, shellfish—such as shrimp, lobster, and crab—are packed with protein and are low in saturated fats, but they also come with hefty amounts of cholesterol. For example, four ounces of shrimp delivers about 25g of protein but about 200g of cholesterol. I usually encourage my patients to limit consumption of shellfish.

Legumes, including beans, peas, and lentils, are good alternatives to animal proteins. These vegetarian proteins contain no cholesterol and are low in fat, high in fiber, and chock-full of nutrients. They are also a good source of soluble and insoluble fiber.

Saturated Fat and Cholesterol Content in Proteins

Protein (per 100g serving)	Saturated Fat (in grams)	Cholesterol (in milligrams)
Beef brisket (1/8-inch fat, braised)	8	107
Beef short ribs (braised)	18	94
Beef (ground, 70% lean meat, broiled)	7	88
Black beans (cooked)	<1	0
Chicken breast (skinless, grilled)	1	104
Crab (Dungeness, cooked)	<1	76
Eggs (scrambled)	3	277
Lamb (1/4-inch fat, roasted)	10	95
Lentils	<1	0
Lobster (northern, cooked)	<1	146
Peas	<1	0
Pork (loin chops, pan-fried)	4	82
Salmon (wild, cooked)	1	71
Shrimp (cooked)	<1	189
Tofu (extra firm)	<1	0
Tuna (bluefin, cooked)	2	49
Turkey (light meat, roasted)	<1	80
Veal (loin, braised)	7	118

Source: USDA Food Composition Databases (numbers have been rounded to the nearest whole number)

GO NUTS

Nuts, when eaten in moderation, can be good for your heart. Nuts pack a powerful nutritional punch, offering good fats, protein, fiber, vitamins, and minerals. Plus, they're cholesterol free. Studies show that eating 6 to 7g of nuts per day decreases total cholesterol and, in particular, LDL by almost 10mg per deciliter. In another study on the Mediterranean diet, eating 30g of nuts per week (15g of walnuts and 7.5g each of almonds and hazelnuts) lowered LDL and triglycerides.

Understand that this doesn't give you free license to polish off a bag of peanuts at the ball game. Take note that 6g to 7g is the equivalent of only about ¼ ounce. That's about seven peanuts, five almonds, four cashews, or three walnut halves. I recommend eating a few nuts a couple times per week for heart health.

DO YOU NEED DIETARY SUPPLEMENTS?

Even if you eat a balanced diet, you may not be getting all the nutrients your body needs for peak heart health. And if you have high cholesterol, you may benefit from taking certain dietary supplements. Be aware that natural substances and supplements may interact with other medications, so be sure to talk to your doctor before taking any supplements.

Fish Oil Supplements

Fish oil supplements are high in omega-3 fatty acids, essential polyunsaturated fats your body needs but can't produce on its own. The only way to get this essential fat is through your food or a dietary supplement. Omega-3 fatty acids are commonly found in fatty fish, such as salmon, trout, tuna, mackerel, and herring. Plant-based foods, including flaxseeds, vegetable oils, and nuts (especially walnuts) are also good sources of omega-3.

Touted for their health benefits, omega-3 fatty acids and fish oil supplements have been at the center of a wealth of scientific research. The research findings so far show these essential fatty acids can:

- Reduce triglyceride levels
- Improve arterial function
- Lower the risk of arrhythmias
- Reduce the risk of sudden cardiac death
- Lower very low-density lipoproteins (VLDL)
- Reduce inflammation
- Lower blood pressure
- Lower heart rate

When combined with statins, they also lower the risk of heart attack and unstable angina, and reduce the likelihood of requiring bypass surgery or stenting to open up blocked arteries.

Omega-3 fatty acids are composed of three compounds:

- *Eicosapentaenoic acid (EPA):* EPA is found mainly in fish.
- *Docosahexaenoic acid (DHA):* Primarily found in fish, DHA may also be present in algae.
- *Alpha-linolenic acid (ALA):* ALA comes from plant sources, such as flaxseed and vegetable oils. Americans tend to consume far more ALA than EPA and DHA, but the benefits of ALA are not nearly as potent as those of EPA and DHA.

Their effects are so well-documented that cardiologists often recommend high doses of fish oil supplements to lower triglycerides. In general, 6g of fish oil per day has proven effective in reducing triglyceride levels. In people with extremely high triglyceride levels, a condition called hypertriglyceridemia, taking 15g per day can result in large reductions in triglycerides.

When looking for a fish oil supplement, be sure to check the amount of EPA and DHA included in each serving. A supplement may claim to provide 1000mg of omega-3 fatty acids per serving, yet EPA and DHA may constitute less than half that amount, with additives making up the rest. Compare nutrition labels and choose one that provides a high amount of EPA and DHA. Minor side effects may include nausea, belching, bad breath, heartburn, rash, nosebleeds, and loose stool.

Phytosterols

Phytosterols, also referred to as plant sterols, are natural compounds found in plants that may lower cholesterol levels. Phytosterols are similar in structure to cholesterol. When you consume them, your digestive system can't tell the difference between the plant sterols and dietary cholesterol. As a result, your digestive system absorbs the plant sterols, which decreases the amount of dietary cholesterol that gets absorbed.

Although existing studies on phytosterols have shown some improvements in cholesterol levels, in particular lowering LDL levels, the data isn't very strong. Additional studies are needed to determine how beneficial plant sterols are in lowering LDL and reducing the risk of CHD. In the meantime, doctors may recommend that patients who need to lower their cholesterol levels take 1g to 3g of phytosterols per day. Common side effects associated with plant sterols include bloating, nausea, diarrhea, and constipation.

Red Yeast Rice

Red yeast rice is a natural compound produced by rice that has been cultured with yeast. It contains monacolin K, a chemically similar enzyme to the active ingredient found in statins, cholesterol-lowering prescription drugs (see Chapter 5). Because of this, red yeast rice can play an important role in reducing cholesterol in some patients. Other potentially beneficial compounds found in red yeast rice include plant sterols, isoflavones, and MUFAs.

This supplement may be recommended as an alternative for people who need to lower their cholesterol but can't take statins due to side effects. Those who are taking statins but still haven't achieved their cholesterol goals may also take red yeast rice. Side effects are generally mild and may include headaches, nausea, and heartburn.

Vitamins

Many of my patients want to know if it's a good idea to take vitamins to compensate for any nutritional shortcomings in their daily diets. Unfortunately, the answer isn't clear. Decades of research on vitamins and antioxidants have produced conflicting findings: Some studies show heart-protecting factors while others produce disappointing results. In general, there is some evidence to support taking a daily multivitamin and a B12 vitamin.

Heart-Harmful or Heart-Healthy?

⊘ Evidence of harm: foods to limit or avoid

 Coconut oil and palm oil are high in saturated fatty acids and raise cholesterol

Eggs have a serum cholesterol-raising effect

Juicing of fruits/vegetables with pulp removal increases caloric concentration*

Southern diets (added fats & oils, fried foods, eggs, organ & processed meats, sugar-sweetened drinks)

⑦ Inconclusive evidence for harm or benefit

Sunflower oil and other liquid vegetable oils

Juicing of fruits/vegetables without pulp removal*

Gluten-containing foods (for people without gluten-related disease)

High-dose antioxidant supplements

⊘ Evidence of benefit: recommended

Extra-virgin olive oil reduces some Cardiovascular Disease outcomes when consumed in moderate quantities

Green leafy vegetables have significant cardio-protective properties when consumed daily

Blueberries and strawberries (>3 servings/week) induce protective antioxidants

Plant-based proteins are significantly more heart healthy than animal proteins

Nuts: 30g serving/day. Portion control is necessary to avoid weight gain. **

* Juicing becomes less of a benefit if calorie intake increases because of caloric concentration with pulp removal.

** Moderate quantities are required to prevent caloric excess.

Freeman, A.M. et al. J am Coll Cardiol. 2017;69(9):1172-87

CHAPTER 10

WEIGHT LOSS FOR CARDIAC PATIENTS

O ne of the most common questions I hear from my patients is, "Do I need to lose weight?" That's what my patient Al asked me during a follow-up appointment after he'd suffered an NSTEMI heart attack and undergone angioplasty and stenting to open up two blocked arteries. Al, a former college football player, was 6 feet 4 inches tall and weighed 250 pounds. I had to break the news to him that his weight fell in the obese category, which increased his risk of coronary events. To reach a healthy weight, he would have to lose about 50 pounds. He was only 51 years old and had a wife and two daughters in college. He told me he wanted to make sure he was around to walk his daughters down the aisle someday. If losing weight would improve his chances of doing that, then he was ready to make changes to his diet.

He asked me which diet he should follow, and I pointed him to several evidence-based eating plans that promote better heart health. I sent him to a nutrition counselor, who helped him choose the one he thought he could stick with long term. After several months of following his new eating plan, Al hit a healthy weight. But the number on the scale wasn't the only one that had improved. Al's lipid profile changed dramatically, with his LDL cholesterol going down by 30 points, his triglycerides dropping by over 50 points, and his HDL level increasing by 15 points. His blood pressure improved and his inflammation biomarker, CRP, dropped into the healthy range. His overall heart-health picture put him in the low-risk category for another coronary event. About five years later, Al got his wish and walked his eldest daughter down the aisle at her wedding.

If you are overweight or obese, losing weight is one of the best things you can do to improve your heart health. Obesity is associated with:

- increased risk of CHD
- abnormal lipid profiles (low HDL, high LDL, high triglycerides, high apo-B)
- thickening of the heart muscle (ventricular hypertrophy)
- coronary arterial dysfunction leading to atherosclerosis

In addition, it raises the risk of Type 2 diabetes, high blood pressure, insulin resistance, obstructive sleep apnea, and metabolic syndrome. The risks associated with obesity are exacerbated if you carry your extra weight around the midsection. Abdominal obesity, also known as visceral fat, is particularly associated with metabolic syndrome. Research shows that people with metabolic syndrome have three times the risk of developing CHD or stroke compared with people who don't have the syndrome.

To determine if you are overweight or obese, know your body mass index (BMI), which is a ratio of weight and height. BMI is broken down into five categories: underweight, healthy weight, overweight, obese, and morbidly obese. The equation to calculate BMI is complicated and involves converting your height into meters and your weight into kilograms. Rather than testing your math skills, you can simply go online to find several BMI calculators. Just plug in your height (in feet and inches) and weight (in pounds), and your BMI will be calculated for you. When you know your number, you can see which weight category you fall into.

Body Mass Index (BMI) Categories

- Underweight: <18.5
- Healthy weight: 18.5-24.9
- Overweight: 25-29.9
- Obese: 30 or higher
- Morbidly obese: 40 or higher

Source: CDC

How much does being overweight or obese affect your heart health? The AHA considers obesity an important risk factor for developing CHD. Research shows that for every five-unit increase in BMI, the risk of coronary events jumps by 29 percent. The risk is seen in both men and women. In the landmark Framingham Heart Study, overweight men had over four times the mortality rate compared with men at an ideal weight. In this study, which followed thousands of people over four decades, overweight was described as being 110 percent of the ideal weight. In another study, women with a BMI over 32 had four times more risk of developing CHD versus women with a BMI less than 19.

Losing weight can lower your risk of CHD by improving your lipid profile, lowering blood pressure, decreasing insulin resistance, decreasing inflammation, and improving the function of your heart muscle and arteries.

To shed pounds, focus your diet on the heart-healthy foods discussed in this chapter, exercise regularly, and practice stress reduction. (Exercise and stress management are covered in greater detail in Chapter 11.) For some people, replacing foods filled with saturated fats, sugar, and sodium with healthier fare may be enough to reduce your weight to a healthy BMI. If necessary, you may also need to lower your daily calorie intake.

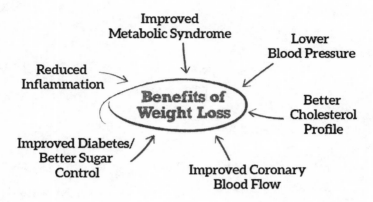

Understanding how many calories you need to consume to reach and maintain your goal weight is an important part of healthy eating. Your individual calorie needs depend primarily on your age, gender, and activity level. For example, a highly active 60-year-old man needs more calories per day than a sedentary woman of the same age. Talk to your doctor to determine your ideal daily calorie intake or see the chart below for an estimate.

Estimated Daily Calorie Needs

Age	Females Activity Level*			Males Activity Level*		
	Sedentary	Moderate	Active	Sedentary	Moderate	Active
18	1,800	2,000	2,400	2,400	2,800	3,200
19-20	2,000	2,200	2,400	2,600	2,800	3,000
21-25	2,000	2,200	2,400	2,400	2,800	3,000
26-30	1,800	2,000	2,400	2,400	2,600	3,000
31-35	1,800	2,000	2,200	2,400	2,600	3,000
36-40	1,800	2,000	2,200	2,400	2,600	2,800

Age	Females Activity Level*			Males Activity Level*		
	Sedentary	Moderate	Active	Sedentary	Moderate	Active
41-45	1,800	2,000	2,200	2,200	2,600	2,800
46-50	1,800	2,000	2,200	2,200	2,400	2,800
51-55	1,600	2,000	2,200	2,200	2,400	2,800
56-60	1,600	2,000	2,200	2,200	2,400	2,600
61-65	1,600	2,000	2,000	2,000	2,400	2,600
66-70	1,600	2,000	2,000	2,000	2,200	2,600
71-75	1,600	2,000	2,000	2,000	2,200	2,600
76 and up	1,600	2,000	2,000	2,000	2,200	2,400

*Activity levels are defined as sedentary (only the physical activities of independent living), moderate (physical activity equivalent to walking 1.5 to 3 miles per day at 3 to 4 miles per hour in addition to independent living), and active (physical activity equivalent to walking over 3 miles per day at 3 to 4 miles per hour in addition to independent living).
Source: USDA Food Patterns

If you are obese or are having trouble losing weight, there is help. Additional weight-loss tools include nutritional counseling, anti-obesity medication, and weight-loss surgery (gastric bypass or banding). Talk with your doctor to determine the best weight-loss plan for you.

HEART-HEALTHY DIETS

Many diets claim to promote heart health, but how do you know which one you should follow? I have found that when my patients try a diet that is too restrictive, too complicated, or that requires dramatic changes, they tend to give up after a few months. Because of this, I steer my patients to eating plans that are easy to follow, allow for a variety of food groups, and can be achieved through small changes. Overall, the best strategy is to adopt a plan you can stick with for the rest of your life. Here, you'll find quick-hit overviews of some of the most popular, evidence-based heart-healthy diets. Work with your doctor to choose the one that suits you best.

Healthy Eating Patterns

INCLUDE:

Vegetables: dark green, red & orange, legumes (beans & peas)

Fruits: especially whole fruits

Grains: half of which are whole grains

Dairy: (fat-free/low-fat) milk, yogurt, cheese, fortified soy drinks

Oils: olive oil, extra-virgin olive oil, some vegetable oils

Proteins: seafood, lean meats, poultry, soy products,
legumes (beans & peas), nuts, seeds

LIMITS: saturated fats and trans fats, added sugars, sodium, eggs

USDA Food Patterns : Healthy U.S.-Style Eating Patterns
(Dietary Guidelines 2015)

American Heart Association and American College of Cardiology Guidelines

The AHA and ACC collaborate with other organizations to develop lifestyle guidelines that promote cardiovascular health. The AHA/ACC guidelines recognize eating a healthy diet as one of the best ways to lower cholesterol and combat CHD. In general, the AHA/ACC plan recommends eating nutrient-dense foods from all food groups while limiting saturated fats, trans fats, sodium, sweets, and red meats.

Within this basic framework, the plan focuses on eating vegetables, fruits, and whole grains. Low-fat or nonfat dairy, skinless poultry, fish, legumes, nuts, and vegetable oils (except tropical oils) are also included. The AHA/ACC guidelines also recognize the importance of maintaining a healthy weight, so check with your doctor to determine your daily calorie needs and stick within those limits.

USDA Food Patterns

Every five years, the U.S. Department of Agriculture (USDA) and the U.S. Department of Health and Human Services (HHS) join together to develop and publish the *Dietary Guidelines for Americans*. This publication reflects the latest science-based findings about food and nutrition and serves as an invaluable resource for healthcare professionals to help their patients make healthy food choices. According to the 2015-2020 *Dietary Guidelines for Americans*, a healthy eating pattern emphasizes nutrient-filled foods and encourages limiting foods that promote disease.

DASH Diet

DASH (Dietary Approaches to Stop Hypertension) was initially created to reduce high blood pressure. However, research shows that in addition to lowering blood pressure, the DASH diet also decreases cholesterol levels and offers cardiovascular protection. This lifelong eating plan focuses on vegetables, fruits, low-fat and nonfat dairy, whole grains, beans, fish, poultry, nuts, and heart-healthy fats. For young, healthy people who aren't at high risk of high blood pressure, the DASH diet limits sodium to less than 2,300mg per day. The daily limit is 1,500mg per day for people who are over age 51, are African-American, or who have:

AHA/ACC Daily Nutrient Breakdown

- 50 percent of calories from carbohydrates
- 20 percent of calories from protein
- Less than 30 percent of calories from fats
- Less than 10 percent of calories from saturated fats
- More than 300mg of polyunsaturated fatty acids
- Less than 3,000mg of sodium (2,400mg, or 1,500mg if you have high blood pressure)
- No more than 2 ounces of alcohol

- high blood pressure
- diabetes
- chronic kidney disease

To follow the DASH diet, check the following guidelines for daily servings allowed, serving sizes, and food recommendations.

DASH Diet Daily Servings

(Number of servings are based on a diet of 2,000 calories per day. Adjust servings based on your individual daily calorie needs.)

Food Group	Servings	1 Serving Size	Recommendations
Whole Grains	7-8 servings per day	1 slice bread 1 ounce dry cereal ½ cup rice or pasta	whole grain bread whole grain oats, cereal brown rice, whole wheat pasta
Vegetables	4-5 servings per day	1 cup raw or green leafy veggies ½ cup cut-up raw or cooked veggies	broccoli, tomatoes, carrots, sweet potatoes, and other veggies
Fruits	4-5 servings per day	1 medium fruit ½ cup fresh/frozen/ canned fruit 4 oz. juice	most fruits except coconuts; leave skin on when possible
Dairy	2-3 servings per day	1 cup skim milk 1 cup low-fat yogurt 1½ oz. part-skim cheese	low-fat, skim, or nonfat

Food Group	Servings	1 Serving Size	Recommendations
Nuts/Seeds, Legumes	4-5 servings per week	1/3 cup nuts 2 tablespoons seeds ½ cup cooked beans/ peas/lentils	almonds, peas, kidney beans, lentils

Animal Protein	2 servings per day	3 oz. lean meat, poultry, fish	lean meats with fat trimmed, white-meat poultry (no skin), fish rich in omega-3; baked, broiled, grilled, roasted, no frying
Eggs	4 servings per week	1 whole egg 2 egg whites 1 fluid oz. egg substitute	soft-boiled, hard-boiled, scrambled, no frying
Fats	2-3 servings per day	1 tablespoon 2 tablespoons salad dressing 1 teaspoon vegetable oil 1 teaspoon soft margarine	olive oil, mayonnaise limit trans fats
Sweets	5 servings per week	1 tablespoon sugar 1 tablespoon jam/jelly ½ cup sorbet 1 cup sweetened lemonade	should be low in fat, such as frozen yogurt, sorbet

Source: DASHdiet.org

Mediterranean Diet

The Mediterranean diet focuses on the foods traditionally eaten in the countries—such as Italy, Greece, and Spain—that border the Mediterranean Sea. A growing body of evidence shows the Mediterranean diet lowers LDL cholesterol and reduces the risk of CHD, stroke, cancer, and other diseases. One study showed that among people at high risk of developing CHD, switching to a Mediterranean diet lowered their risk of heart attacks, strokes,

Mediterranean Diet Intake Recommendations

- High intake: fruits, vegetables, whole grains, legumes, and nuts
- Moderate intake: fish, poultry, and healthy fats
- Low intake: dairy products, red meat, processed meats, and sweets

and cardiovascular-related deaths by about 30 percent.

On this heart-healthy plan, you're also encouraged to enjoy wine in moderation, as long as it is consumed with meals. About 30 to 35 percent of your total daily calories should come from fat, with an emphasis on polyunsaturated fats like olive oil that are high in omega-3 fatty acids. Saturated fats, however, should be limited to 9 to 10 percent of your total daily calories. The fat allowances for the Mediterranean diet are slightly higher than those recommended by the AHA/ACC. Ask your doctor how much fat you should be eating.

One reason the Mediterranean diet is so beneficial is that it is so high in fiber. On this diet, you should aim for 27 to 37g of fiber per day. This includes fruits and vegetables, as well as whole grain breads and pastas and legumes.

Another important aspect of the Mediterranean diet is *how* you eat. Enjoying meals with friends and family is one of the foundations of this eating style.

Plant-Based Diets

For a variety of reasons—better health, weight loss, environmentalism, concern for animal welfare, economics, or religion—plant-based diets are gaining in popularity. There are several types of plant-based diets, ranging from those that exclude all animal proteins to those that include eggs, dairy, and even an occasional serving of meat, poultry, or fish.

Worldwide, there are about 375 million vegetarians. In the U.S., approximately 8 million adults are vegetarians, and of those, about 3.7 million are vegan, according to a Harris Poll conducted for the Vegetarian Resource Group. Flexitarianism is a relatively new concept that is on the rise. People who aren't ready or willing to commit fully to a vegetarian or vegan diet but still want the health benefits may find it easier to adopt this dietary approach.

The medical community has known about the health benefits of plant-based diets for many years. Studies have revealed that people living in Okinawa, Japan; the highlands of Papua, New Guinea; and central Africa have little to no cardiovascular disease. In large part, this is credited to the fact that their diets consist mainly of plant-based foods.

Types of Plant-Based Diets

- **Ovo-lacto vegetarians:** diet avoids most animal products but includes eggs and dairy

- **Lacto vegetarians:** diet avoids most animal products but includes dairy

- **Ovo vegetarians:** diet avoids most animal products but includes eggs

- **Vegans:** diet avoids all animal products

- **Flexitarian:** diet is mostly vegetarian with occasional animal proteins

Caldwell B. Esselstyn Jr., M.D., director of the Cardiovascular Disease Prevention and Reversal Program at the Cleveland Clinic Wellness Institute and author of "Prevent and Reverse Heart Disease," has studied the cardiovascular health effects of whole food, plant-based nutrition since the 1990s. His research concluded that adhering to this type of diet reduces the risk of major coronary events, including heart attack, stroke, and death. In one of Esselstyn's trials, people who had undergone cardiac interventions, such as bypass surgery or angioplasty, were followed for nearly four years. Among those who stuck to the plant-based nutrition program, 99.4 percent avoided further major coronary events.

Another notable cardiologist, Dean Ornish, M.D., director of the Preventive Medicine Research Institute and author of "Dr. Dean Ornish's Program for Reversing Heart Disease" and several other books, began reporting his findings on plant-based nutrition and cardiovascular health in the 1990s. His body of work has shown that comprehensive lifestyle changes—including stress management and a low-fat vegetarian diet without added oils—may slow, stop, or even reverse CHD.

Following on the heels of these pioneers, many other researchers have put plant-based diets to the test. The results show that this style of eating protects against CHD. Several mechanisms are at work. Green leafy vegetables—such as arugula, Swiss chard, celery, collard greens, kale, and spinach—increase production of nitric oxide, which reduces the stiffness of coronary arteries. Green vegetables—such as asparagus, broccoli, green beans, parsley, kale, spinach, and zucchini—are rich in carotenoids, which have antioxidant and anti-inflammatory properties. In addition, green vegetables increase insulin sensitivity, which leads to better blood-sugar control and reduces the incidence of diabetes.

In spite of all these benefits, some people are concerned that a plant-based diet won't provide adequate protein. Rest assured that there are many meat-free protein options. Protein-rich vegetarian foods include legumes, which contain almost as much protein as animal foods but without the fat or sodium. For example, one cup of cooked lentils provides about 18g of protein. Even better, lentils don't have any fat or sodium. By comparison, 6 ounces of steak may contain 42g of protein, but it also comes with 12g of artery-clogging fat. You may be surprised to learn that some grains and green leafy vegetables are also good sources of protein. Use the following chart to help you create heart-healthy vegetarian meals that are rich in protein.

Protein-Rich Vegetarian Foods

	Serving Size	Protein Content
Tempeh	1 cup	31g
Tofu	1 cup	20g
Lentils (cooked)	1 cup	18g
Beans (black, cooked)	1 cup	15g
Peas (cooked)	1 cup	8g
Quinoa (cooked)	1 cup	8g
Soy milk	1 cup	8g
Almonds	¼ cup	5g
Chia seeds	1 oz.	5g
Broccoli	1 cup	3g
Spinach	1 cup	1g

Source: USDA

FOR MORE INFORMATION ON HEALTHY EATING

This chapter provides only highlights of some of the most evidence-based, heart-healthy eating plans. If you would like additional details on these diets, check the Resources section of this book for links to additional information.

CHAPTER 11

MOVE MORE, STRESS LESS, AND TAME DEPRESSION

In addition to adopting a heart-smart diet and maintaining a healthy weight, participating in regular physical exercise, practicing stress management, and keeping depression at bay can go a long way in improving your cardiovascular health. Indeed, they are an integral part of any cardiac rehabilitation program following a heart attack, angioplasty, coronary artery bypass graft (CABG) surgery, or other coronary event.

Over the past 20-plus years, I've helped thousands of patients complete cardiac rehab and boost their heart health. Angela is no exception. A 62-year-old high-powered attorney, she came to my office following an acute coronary syndrome (ACS) episode that resulted in angioplasty and stenting of one of her arteries. As I do with all my patients diagnosed with CHD, I asked her about her exercise habits, daily stress levels, and any signs of depression. She said she didn't feel depressed but admitted she was a bit of a couch potato and said her stress was through the roof. She always felt frazzled at the end of the day.

I told her if she could move more and stress less, she could improve her heart health and reduce the risk of future coronary events. Because of her busy schedule, I recommended she ease into physical activity. She started walking for about 10 minutes three days a week. To her surprise, she enjoyed an evening walk after a stressful day and found it calming. Over time, she gradually increased her activity level. Within six months, Angela was taking a 30-minute brisk walk almost every evening and then doing some deep breathing and yoga stretches when she finished.

At the end of her day, she felt refreshed, not frazzled. And she felt like she could handle the daily stressors at work better. Combined with medication therapy to treat her cholesterol levels, the new activity also improved her cardiac function. Her treadmill tests showed better cardiovascular fitness and a lower heart rate. Seven years later, her tests show she's at low risk of a coronary event.

While integrating physical activity and stress management into your daily routine and treating depression can reduce your risk of heart disease, you don't have to become a bulked-up bodybuilder, a long-distance runner, or a Zen master to see results. Check out the simple guidelines in this chapter for a road map to get you on the path to better cardiovascular health. Your heart will thank you for it.

MOVE MORE

The science is clear: Inactivity is an important risk factor for premature CHD. The good news is that whether you've already experienced a heart attack or ACS episode or you're at high risk of CHD, physical activity can improve your cardiovascular health. In people diagnosed with CHD, physical activity is associated with a lower incidence of death from all causes. According to decades of research, the benefits of physical activity include:

- Minimizes the risk of CHD
- Improves existing CHD
- Enhances blood flow
- Boosts the heart's working capacity

- Lowers resting heart rate
- Helps with weight loss/weight management
- Reduces blood pressure
- Improves blood sugar control
- Increases HDL
- Lowers LDL
- Improves overall muscle function (general muscles, not the heart muscle)
- Improves oxygen delivery to body tissues
- Decreases the frequency of angina episodes

Both men and women experience these benefits. For example, men over 65 who walk 2 miles a day are less likely to die than those who walk just 1 mile. And women who engage in brisk walking—even if they don't become active until later in life—are less likely to experience a coronary event.

Measuring Your Fitness Level

How important is physical activity to your overall health? In people with CHD it's a strong predictor of longevity—the higher your cardiac fitness level, the lower your risk of dying. To determine your fitness level, doctors evaluate something called your peak exercise capacity, which is basically your maximum exertion level before you go breathless. This is usually evaluated during a stress test, which is also known as a treadmill test. (You can read more about stress tests in Chapter 4.)

As you exercise, your cardiovascular system delivers oxygen to your muscles, and your muscles extract that oxygen and transition it into the bloodstream. This keeps you breathing efficiently during physical activity. Your oxygen delivery and uptake cycle has a limit, however. It's your body's way of telling you to slow down when you're exercising at your highest intensity. Think of sprinting uphill, pedaling as fast as you can on your bike, or taking those last few steps on the stair climber. If you can sustain an intensity level for only about 10 to 15 seconds before going breathless, you've hit your peak exercise capacity.

Physical exertion is measured in something called metabolic equivalents, or METs, which determine your fitness level. The more intense the physical activity, the higher the METs. Sitting quietly, for example, is equal to 1 MET; walking at 3 miles per hour correlates to 4 METs; jogging at 6 miles per hour is over 6 METs; and running at 8 miles per hour clocks in at over 13 METs. The higher the number of METs when you reach your peak exercise capacity, the greater your fitness level. Active athletes can have a peak exercise capacity as high as 18 METs. For nonathletic but active, healthy middle-aged men, the average is 10 METs, about 2 METs higher than the average for women in the same age range.

If your peak exercise capacity is lower than average, take heart. You can improve it by engaging in physical exercise on a regular basis. I see this often in my practice. I've seen patients who could only walk very slowly for a few minutes on a treadmill go from fitness levels of less than 3 METs to over 10 METs. The key to improvement is to increase your efforts gradually under your doctor's guidance.

How Much Exercise Do You Need?

To improve your heart health, you don't need to sprint 10 miles a day or spend hours in the gym lifting heavy weights. In fact, research shows that you can see a reduction in CHD with as little as:

- running: one hour or more per week
- rowing: one hour or more per week
- brisk walking: at least 30 minutes a day
- lifting weights: 30 minutes or more per week

A number of organizations offer guidelines for the amount of exercise you should get. Their recommendations are based on intensity

Light-Intensity Activities

- Walking slowly (shopping, walking around the house or office)
- Preparing food
- Light housework (washing dishes, dusting)
- Biking slowly (less than 5 mph)
- Stretching
- Sitting at the computer
- Fishing
- Golf (using a cart)
- Desk jobs

levels—using METs—and broken down into three categories:

- light: <3 METs
- moderate: 3-6 METs
- vigorous: >6 METs

In general, when you're engaging in light-intensity activities, your breathing and heart rate don't increase and you don't break into a sweat. With moderate-intensity exercise you'll start to perspire, your heart rate will speed up, and your breathing will deepen, but you'll still be able to carry on a conversation. When you kick it up a notch into vigorous activities, you'll start sweating in a few minutes, you'll take quick and deep breaths, your heart will beat even faster, and you'll only be able to utter brief words or phrases.

American Heart Association and American College of Cardiology Recommendations

For the prevention of CHD—whether you've already been diagnosed or are simply at risk of it—the AHA and ACC recommend at least 30 minutes of moderate-intensity exercise five to seven days per week. Depending on your individual condition, however, you may need to exercise at a lower intensity for less time. For example, if you are in the early stages of recovery after a heart attack or ACS episode, start slowly and build up to the recommended intensity and duration.

If you have been diagnosed with chronic stable angina, your doctor will likely perform an exercise test to evaluate your fitness level and determine how much exercise is ideal for you. Many people with chronic stable angina are able to meet the general recommendations of at least 30 minutes of moderate-intensity exercise five to seven days per week.

People diagnosed with CHD who engage in moderate- or vigorous-intensity activities experience lower death rates. This has been shown with the following types and duration of activity:

- recreational/nonsporting activities: over four hours per week
- walking: over 40 minutes per day
- moderate to heavy gardening: 30 minutes or more per day

U.S. Department of Health & Human Services and CDC Recommendations

HHS in conjunction with the CDC recommends moderate- or vigorous-intensity activity in addition to strength training that works all the muscles in the body (legs, arms, shoulders, back, chest, core) as follows:

Moderate-Intensity Activities

- Brisk walking
- Hiking/walking uphill
- Slow jogging (up to 6 mph)
- Biking (5-9 mph)
- Yoga
- Weight training
- Active housework (vacuuming)
- Recreational swimming
- Golf (carrying clubs)
- Tennis (doubles)
- Jobs that require standing or walking

- 150 minutes of moderate-intensity activity per week
- at least two days of strength training per week

OR

- 75 minutes of vigorous-intensity activity per week
- at least two days of strength training per week

OR

Vigorous-Intensity Activities

- Running (over 6 mph)
- Race walking (over 4.5 mph)
- Mountain climbing
- Backpacking
- Biking (over 10 mph)
- Jumping rope
- Jumping jacks
- Tennis (singles)
- Jobs that require heavy lifting

- an equivalent mix of moderate-intensity and vigorous-intensity activity per week
- at least two days of strength training per week

Within these recommendations, there is a lot of flexibility. It's up to you to decide how you want to split up your workout sessions. Just remember, you need to move for at least 10 minutes at a time to reap the benefits. For example, to reach 150 minutes of moderate-intensity activity, you might break it up into 30-minute sessions five times a week. Or you could do three 10-minute segments a day five times a week. The choice is up to you.

Minimum Recommended Exercise for Healthy Adults

Moderate-intensity aerobic exercise for 150 min/week AND Muscle-strengthening exercises at least 2 days/week	OR	Vigorous-intensity aerobic exercise for 75 min/week AND Muscle-strengthening activites at least 2 days/week	OR	Equivalent mix of moderate- & vigorous-intensity aerobic exercise AND Muscle-strengthening activities at least 2 days/week

U.S. Department of Health & Human Services and Centers for Disease Control & Prevention

Getting Started: Take It Easy

The recommended amounts of exercise may seem daunting at first. If you're feeling this way, follow the strategy I use with my patients. I generally encourage them to take a gentle approach to exercise, especially if they are new to a fitness program. Start with 10 or 15 minutes a few times a week, and always keep in mind that some activity is better than no activity. Find an activity that you enjoy—walking, hiking, playing tennis, dancing, swimming—and you will be far more likely to stick with it for the long run.

STRESS LESS AND TAME DEPRESSION

As you have seen in this book, your mental health plays a role in your heart health. Numerous studies have linked depression and stressful events—such as a job loss or the death of a loved one—with sudden cardiac death and heart attacks. Stress and depression raise the risk of CHD in a variety of ways.

Mental stress can lead to a number of physical factors associated with heightened risk of CHD:

- arterial dysfunction
- platelet activation (causing blood to become more sticky and increasing clot formation)
- inflammation
- impaired nitric oxide (prevents arteries from dilating and affects blood flow, causing more chest pain and leading to more heart attacks and death)
- angina (leads to reduced coronary blood flow)

Depression has been linked to the following physical factors that contribute to the premature development of CHD:

- damage to the inner lining of arteries
- platelet abnormalities

- angina
- inflammation

Both stress and depression are also associated with a tendency to engage in behaviors that put you at greater risk of CHD:

- smoking
- physical inactivity
- drinking too much alcohol
- overeating
- inadequate sleep

These behaviors also take a physical toll, contributing to high blood pressure, high cholesterol, diabetes, and other conditions that raise the risk of CHD.

Treating Stress and Depression

The consequences of stress and depression are so strong that cardiologists routinely screen CHD patients for depression and include stress management as part of cardiac rehab programs.

If you're diagnosed with depression, which is present in one in three heart attack victims, there are many treatment options available. On a positive note, some of the same lifestyle recommendations that protect heart health may also improve depression. For example, physical activity, which boosts the production of feel-good chemicals known as endorphins, has been shown to reduce symptoms of depression. In addition, some studies suggest that eating a heart-healthy diet that includes foods high in omega-3 fatty acids can help keep depression at bay. Other lifestyle changes that can boost your mood include getting enough sleep, staying in touch with family and friends, meditating, and getting some sunshine every day.

If necessary, your doctor may prescribe antidepressant medications. Taking these medications is critical for some people and can reduce the risk of mortality. Note that some older types of antidepressant medications, such as tricyclic or MAOI drugs, are used with caution in people with CHD due to the risk of heart arrhythmia. Newer medications to treat depression don't have these negative heart rhythm side effects. Talk to your doctor about the best medication for your individual condition.

If chronic stress is plaguing you, the keys are to reduce the stressors in your life and find better ways to handle daily stresses. Reducing stress shows almost immediate physiological improvements. For example, in moments of heightened stress, your body's fight-or-flight response kicks into action, causing your heart rate to accelerate and your breathing to become more shallow, reducing oxygen consumption. Relaxation, on the other hand, activates the parasympathetic nervous system, which shuts off that fight-or-flight response by slowing your heart rate, deepening your breathing, and increasing oxygen consumption.

There are many natural ways to relieve stress. Physical activity and eating a heart-healthy diet can help calm stress. Relying on your family and friends, getting enough sleep, and doing meditation or deep-breathing exercises are other ways to soothe stress. In some cases, prescription medications, such as muscle relaxants, may be prescribed.

If you're taking part in a cardiac rehab program, you'll learn about these and possibly other lifestyle changes and medications that may help you fight stress and depression. Sometimes just knowing there is hope for relief can be a great comfort to you and can begin the healing process.

CHAPTER 12

QUIT SMOKING

About a decade ago, I performed angioplasty and stenting on a 61-year-old woman named Rachel. When I saw her in my office for follow-up and ongoing care, I asked her about her lifestyle habits. She admitted she had smoked a pack of cigarettes a day since she was 15. I let her know that smoking contributes to the development of CHD and emphasized that this link is especially strong in women. In fact, female smokers are 25 percent more likely to develop CHD than their male counterparts. I added that continuing to smoke after being diagnosed with CHD, and especially after stenting or bypass surgery, increases the likelihood of requiring a repeat procedure. Even worse, it raises the risk of death from a cardiac event. Usually, when I share this fact with my patients who smoke, it's enough to get them to consider quitting.

Rachel immediately vowed to kick her lifelong habit. I prescribed smoking cessation medication that makes smoking less rewarding and reduces withdrawal symptoms and pointed her to some nicotine replacement products she could use. She opted for a patch that delivers continuous nicotine as well as gum that she could chew whenever she got a strong craving for a cigarette. I also recommended a counseling program that would help keep her on track. In the first few months, she "cheated" several times and thought about giving up on trying to quit. The counselor helped keep her motivated to stick with her resolve. About sixth months later, Rachel was able to stop taking the medication and tossed away the patch and gum. Now, 10 years later, she still hasn't picked up a cigarette, and her cardiovascular health has greatly improved.

For Rachel, quitting smoking was the No. 1 lifestyle change she could make to reduce her risk of heart attack and death. If you're a smoker, it should be your top priority, too. Fortunately, there are many treatment options to help you kick the habit for good.

THE SMOKING-CHD CONNECTION

Did you know that smoking just one cigarette a day increases the risk of CHD and heart attack? Not surprisingly, the risk factor rises with the number of cigarettes smoked. In people who smoke at least 20 cigarettes a day, the incidence of heart attack increases sixfold in women and threefold in men. And people who smoke 40 or more cigarettes a day? They are at the highest risk.

Why is smoking so bad for your heart? It ramps up the progression of atherosclerosis by 50 percent, leading to increases in plaque, blockages, heart attack, and death. Even people who are exposed to secondhand smoke are hit by the harmful effects of the habit, experiencing a 20 percent increase in the atherosclerotic process. Smoking is detrimental to cardiovascular health in many more ways, including:

- adverse effects on lipids (higher LDL and triglycerides, lower HDL)
- higher insulin resistance
- damage from free radicals leading to higher LDL

- parasympathetic increase in heart rate
- clamping of arteries and decrease in blood flow
- the carbon monoxide in smoke leads to high levels of carboxyhemoglobin, which results in less oxygen being transported by the blood
- increased inflammation
- blood cells become more sticky
- increased clotting
- activation of platelets
- reduces elasticity of aorta, causing stiffening and trauma to this vessel
- prevents coronary arteries from expanding, reducing arterial flow and increasing chest pain
- temporary increase in heart rate and blood pressure

Cigars, Pipes, and Electronic Cigarettes

If you smoke cigars, pipes, or e-cigarettes, you may be under the impression that your smoking or "vaping" habit isn't harmful to your health. Many smokers believe cigars and pipes are safe because there's less inhalation compared with cigarettes. And people assume e-cigarettes are harmless because they're smokeless. These are dangerous myths.

Scientific evidence shows that these products increase the risk of CHD; however, the research isn't clear on the mechanisms at work. What we do know is that smoking more than four cigars per day is equivalent to puffing away on 10 cigarettes. Even if you don't inhale with cigars and pipes, you are still inhaling the smoke that's released. And although it's true that e-cigarettes don't burn tobacco, they still deliver nicotine into your system. Cigars, pipes, and e-cigarettes pose additional health risks. For example, cigars contain carcinogens and are associated with an increased risk of lung cancer, abnormalities in the gastrointestinal tract, and emphysema.

THE BENEFITS OF QUITTING SMOKING

The benefits of kicking the smoking habit are undeniable. Just look at the case of Olmstead County, Minnesota. In 2002, the county implemented an ordinance requiring all restaurants to go smoke-free. Five years later, the ordinance expanded to make all workplaces smoke-free zones. A scientific study published in 2012 looked at the number of heart attacks and incidences of sudden cardiac death in the 18 months before and after the enactment of the ordinances. The results were astonishing. The creation of smoke-free workplaces lowered the incidence of heart attacks by 33 percent and sudden cardiac deaths by 17 percent. These impressive statistics show what a dramatic benefit it can be to go smoke-free.

On an individual level, giving up smoking results in about a 17 percent reduction in heart attacks and lowers the risk of being admitted to the hospital with a coronary event by about 40 percent. Quitting triggers a reversal of all the detrimental cardiovascular effects of smoking, and some of these changes begin almost immediately. For example, after smoking your last cigarette, it takes only about 20 minutes for your heart rate to drop back into a normal range and about 12 hours for carbon monoxide levels in the blood to normalize.

GETTING THE HELP YOU NEED TO QUIT SMOKING

Ask anyone who has quit smoking and they'll probably tell you it was one of the hardest things they've ever done. Why is it so hard to quit? The nicotine in cigarettes is highly addictive. When you take a drag on a cigarette, nicotine rushes into your bloodstream and makes its way to your brain within 10 seconds. The nicotine binds to receptors in the brain, which sparks the release of a feel-good brain chemical called dopamine that promotes feelings of pleasure, relaxation, and improved concentration. This mood boost doesn't last, however, and as the effects of nicotine wear off, you start to crave it again. Over time, the brain rewires itself and you need more and more nicotine to achieve the same feeling.

TREATMENT OF
Nicotine Withdrawal Syndrome

Behavioral Counseling from:	Pharmacologic Treatments:	Other Treatments:
- Primary Care - Cardiology Clinic - Smoking Cessation Program	- Nicotine Replacement Patches, Lozenges, Gum, Inhaler, Nasal Spray - Prescription Medications Varenicline/Chantix, Bupropion/Zyban	- Acupuncture - Hypnosis - E-Cigarettes

Trying to quit smoking comes with tough withdrawal symptoms, including mood changes, insomnia, irritability, difficulty concentrating, restlessness, an increase in appetite, and weight gain. Withdrawal symptoms peak in the first three days and then subside in three to four weeks. Many smokers can't get past the withdrawal phase even though they want to quit.

Two-thirds of smokers claim they want to quit, but less than one-third of them seek help in the process. This is too bad because there are several treatment options—counseling programs, nicotine replacement therapy, and medications—to help you kick the habit. With optimal treatment, 25 to 35 percent of people succeed in quitting smoking in six months or more. The best treatment plan for you depends on your degree of nicotine dependence. In general, the more you smoke, the more treatment you'll need. If you're concerned about the cost involved, rest assured that many health insurance plans cover smoking cessation treatment.

Counseling Programs

Counseling programs provide support in your efforts to quit smoking. With these programs, you'll discover tips, strategies, and resources to help you navigate the process—learning how to identify and avoid the triggers that make you crave a cigarette, ways to make it through the withdrawal period, and proven approaches to prevent relapse. Along the way, counselors will help you work through your individual challenges. These programs take many forms, including individual and group counseling, and can be conducted in person, over the phone, via text, or through a website. Research shows that participating in counseling increases your chances of successfully quitting smoking, especially when combined with cessation medication.

Nicotine Replacement Therapy

Nicotine replacement therapy (NRT) products offer small doses of nicotine to help you manage your cravings and reduce physical withdrawal symptoms as you try to quit smoking. Many studies show that you are twice as likely to be successful in your attempt to quit smoking if you use nicotine patches, gum, nasal sprays, inhalers, or lozenges. With my patients, I have found that using two NRT agents, such as a patch and gum, can be more effective than relying on a single agent. NRT is only part of a comprehensive plan to quit smoking. Combining it with medication and counseling can be even more effective.

Some NRT products require a prescription, while others can be purchased over the counter. Before you rush to the drugstore to pick up some gum or lozenges, however, be aware that these products come in different dosages and strengths. The right amount for you depends on how many cigarettes you smoke per day. For example, if you're a heavy smoker, you'll need to start with a higher dosage than a light smoker. Most of these products are taken

What Kind of Smoker Are You?

- **Light smoker:** less than 10 cigarettes per day

- **Moderate smoker:** more than 10 cigarettes per day but less than a pack a day

- **Heavy smoker:** a pack a day or more

Source: American Cancer Society

for several weeks or months. As time passes, you can taper down the dosage until you stop using the products. Talk to your doctor to determine the ideal dosage to help you quit smoking.

NRT is safe to use if you have CHD, unstable angina, and even if you have had an ACS episode or heart attack. In fact, these products are sometimes used in people who are in the hospital with ACS or heart attack. When it comes to heart health, there are some misconceptions about NRT. You may hear that it causes narrowing of arteries, stickiness, and an increased heart rate. Don't let these myths dissuade you from using these products to help you quit smoking. NRT does cause a gradual rise in heart rate, but it does not promote stickiness or blockages in the arteries.

For best results, avoid drinking coffee and carbonated drinks when using NRT because they reduce nicotine absorption. There are some side effects associated with NRT products, including nausea, intestinal pain, diarrhea, headache, and local irritation. It's important to understand that although these products contain nicotine, they don't have the other harmful chemicals found in cigarettes and they don't cause cancer.

Patches

The nicotine patch, which was invented in 1984, is credited with helping millions of people quit smoking. Patches are available with or without a prescription. Applied directly to the skin, the patch delivers a continuous dose of nicotine. Available by prescription and over the counter, these transdermal patches come in a variety of strengths. Using nicotine patches is easy. You simply affix a new patch every morning or every night to a clean, dry area of your skin—such as your arm, chest, or back—where there is relatively little hair.

People who smoke more than 10 cigarettes a day are usually prescribed a 10-week course with tapering dosages as follows:

- **Weeks 1-6:** 21mg per day
- **Weeks 7-8:** 14mg per day
- **Weeks 9-10:** 7mg per day

People who smoke up to 10 cigarettes a day are recommended to follow an eight-week course with the following dosages:

- **Weeks 1-6:** 14mg per day
- **Weeks 7-8:** 7mg per day

Gum

Introduced in the 1980s, nicotine gum is a short-acting NRT product that can calm cravings. At first, you typically need to chew one piece of gum every one to two hours. Over time, you will be encouraged to chew fewer pieces of gum each day. Be sure to avoid chewing more than 24 pieces in a day. For best results, wait at least 15 minutes after a meal before popping a piece in your mouth.

Nicotine gum comes in many familiar flavors—including spearmint, fruit, and cinnamon—so you should be able to find a flavor you like. However, chewing nicotine gum isn't the same as chewing regular gum. It is recommended that you adopt what doctors call a "chew and park" approach. This means you chew the gum until the taste of nicotine appears, then you "park" it between your cheek and gums. Simply let the gum rest there until the nicotine taste disappears, then chew it again. Continue repeating this cycle for a total of 30 minutes, then discard the gum.

Available over the counter, nicotine gum comes in two strengths: 2mg and 4mg of nicotine. If you smoke more than 25 cigarettes a day or if you smoke within the first 30 minutes of waking up in the morning, choose the 4mg dose. If you smoke fewer than 10 cigarettes a day or you typically don't smoke your first cigarette until more than 30 minutes after waking up, opt for the 2mg dose. Stop using nicotine gum after 12 weeks.

- **Weeks 1-6:** One piece of gum every 1-2 hours
- **Weeks 7-8:** One piece of gum every 2-4 hours
- **Weeks 9-10:** One piece of gum every 4-8 hours

Lozenges
Nicotine lozenges are small tablets that resemble hard candy. Like nicotine gum, they offer a temporary dose of nicotine to help curb cravings. When you start using lozenges, take one every one to two hours a day, making sure not to consume more than 20 lozenges a day. Just pop a lozenge in your mouth and let it dissolve, which may take about 20 to 30 minutes. Don't chew the lozenges and always wait at least 15 minutes after eating before taking one.

Lozenges are available in 2mg and 4mg strengths. Heavy smokers and those who smoke within the first hour of waking should start with 4mg and taper down over several weeks. Light smokers and those who can wait longer than 30 minutes before lighting up in the morning should start with 2mg. Over time, use fewer lozenges per day. Lozenges should not be used for more than 12 weeks.

- **Weeks 1-6:** One lozenge every 1-2 hours
- **Weeks 7-8:** One lozenge every 2-4 hours
- **Weeks 9-10:** One lozenge every 4-8 hours

Inhalers

Nicotine inhalers are the only NRT product that mimics the action of smoking, which makes it a good option for people who miss the ritual of smoking. If you love holding a cigarette in your hand, bringing it to your mouth, and taking a puff, you may want to consider using an inhaler to help you quit. Approved by the USDA in 1998, inhalers are available without a prescription at your local drug store. Compared with other NRT products, they deliver a higher initial boost of nicotine to the bloodstream.

Inhalers come with several cartridges. Each cartridge lasts for about 20 minutes or 400 puffs. However, you don't have to finish the cartridge in one sitting. You can puff until your craving subsides—whether that's five, 10, or 15 minutes—and save the rest for later. When you've finished inhaling a cartridge, discard it and replace it with a new one. Don't use more than 16 cartridges in a single day and stop using the inhaler after six months.

- **Weeks 1-12:** 6 to 16 cartridges per day
- **Weeks 13-24:** gradually reduce the number of cartridges

Sprays

Available with a doctor's prescription, nicotine sprays are liquids that you spray into your nose. These sprays deliver peak nicotine levels in the first 10 minutes, then gradually wear off. That initial burst of nicotine is higher than what you get from oral agents, such as gum and lozenges. It is recommended that you start with about one to two sprays per hour. Make sure you don't exceed the maximum dose of 10 sprays per hour. Nasal sprays may cause some minor side effects, including nasal irritation, sneezing, or rhinitis.

- **Weeks 1-12:** 1 to 2 sprays per hour
- **Weeks 13-24:** gradually reduce the number of sprays per day

MEDICATIONS

Prescription drugs, which help reduce cravings and withdrawal symptoms, have been shown to improve your chances of quitting smoking. Medications can be used alone, but they are more effective when used in combination with NRT and counseling. Talk to your doctor to see if medication is right for you.

Varenicline

Available by prescription only, varenicline (brand name Chantix) is a medication that reduces the rewarding effects of smoking and minimizes the symptoms of withdrawal. In your body, this is achieved by blocking nicotine from binding to the receptors in the brain that lead to the release of dopamine. In one study, varenicline was found to be more effective at six months than other cessation medication, the nicotine patch, or a placebo.

For best results, start taking varenicline about one week prior to your "quit day" when you will stop smoking cigarettes. It is generally recommended that you take this medication for 12 weeks or more to prevent relapse. The typical dosage is as follows:

- **Days 1-3:** ½mg per day
- **Days 4-8:** ½mg twice per day for 4 days
- **Day 9-Week 12:** 1mg twice per day

Take the medication with food and an 8-ounce glass of water. Side effects that may occur while taking varenicline include nausea, vomiting, sleep disturbances, abnormal dreams, headache, gas, constipation, changes in taste, skin rashes, mood changes, and heart and blood vessel problems (in people who already have these conditions). Note that using this medication is considered safe for people with CHD. If you experience side effects, your doctor can lower your dosage. If you notice any severe mood changes or suicidal thoughts, stop taking the medication and contact your doctor.

Bupropion

The prescription drug bupropion (brand names Wellbutrin and Zyban) decreases cravings and withdrawal symptoms, but the mechanisms behind this ability are not well known. The drug doesn't act on the brain's nicotine receptors the way other cessation medication does. Bupropion is also commonly prescribed to treat depression, but its antidepressant quality doesn't explain how it helps people stop smoking. You don't have to have depression for this drug to help you quit smoking, but it can be especially useful for those with the mood disorder. The typical recommended dosage for bupropion is as follows:

- **Days 1-3:** 150mg per day
- **Day 4-Week 12:** 150mg twice a day

About one to two weeks after you start taking the medication, your physician will ask you for a follow-up phone call to see how you're doing. Note that about 20 to 25 percent of people relapse while taking bupropion, with most relapses occurring in the first three months after quitting. If you relapse, keep taking the medication, try using NRT to curb cravings, and rely on support from counseling. You can continue taking bupropion for one year or longer. An added benefit of bupropion is that it has been found to prevent the weight gain that is commonly experienced when people quit smoking.

The most common side effects associated with this medication are dry mouth and insomnia. Other side effects include nausea, dizziness, anxiety, constipation, trouble concentrating, skin rashes, and tremors. Bupropion is safe in people with CHD, but it is not recommended for people with seizures.

Alternative Treatments

A growing number of smokers are turning to alternative treatments, such as acupuncture and hypnosis, to help them quit. Some people add natural therapies to their mix of medication, NRT, and counseling in an effort to cover all the bases. Others can't tolerate prescription drugs or NRT products due to side effects or other conditions. The research on these natural therapies isn't strong. Acupuncture has been shown to have some benefits, but it is not as effective as medications or NRT. As for hypnosis, there are many anecdotal stories about its effectiveness, but there is insufficient data to recommend it.

FINAL THOUGHTS ON QUITTING SMOKING

As I mentioned earlier in this chapter, quitting smoking is the No. 1 thing smokers can do to improve heart health. I understand how hard it can be, but I hope you will be encouraged to know that I have seen many of my patients who were lifelong heavy smokers succeed at quitting. Some of them experienced relapses along the way, and you may, too. If you do relapse, just do your best to get back on track. Take advantage of the quitting-smoking therapies described in this chapter, and if you need some immediate encouragement or support, call 1-800-QUIT-NOW to speak to a counselor (note: hours of operation and services vary by state).

CONCLUSION

I hope the information in this book has helped you gain a better understanding of CHD and the many things you can do to take charge of your health, lower your risk of CHD, and prevent future heart attacks. The medical community is continuously making strides in the treatment of CHD, and new procedures and breakthrough medications are on the horizon. To make sure you are receiving the most advanced treatments for your individual needs, work closely with your doctor. Together, as a team, you can find the best treatment options to keep your heart healthy for years to come.

RESOURCES

American Heart Association

www.heart.org/HEARTORG/

This voluntary health organization is dedicated to fighting heart disease and stroke. The website provides a wealth of information and tools to help you understand coronary heart disease, what causes it, and how to prevent it. You can find guidelines on healthy living and an online support network.

CardioSmart

www.cardiosmart.org

This patient education site of the American College of Cardiology (http://www.acc.org/) offers information on heart basics, heart conditions, treatments, and healthy living. You can also join the free CardioSmart online program to set health goals and track your progress. The site also features a comprehensive risk assessment so you can gauge your risk of coronary heart disease.

MedlinePlus

https://medlineplus.gov/

A website from the National Institutes of Health, MedlinePlus offers reliable information about many health conditions, including coronary heart disease. You can learn about conditions, treatment options, prescription drugs and supplements, lifestyle changes, and more. The site also features an extensive video library, interactive calculators, and quizzes.

National Heart, Lung, and Blood Institute

www.nhlbi.nih.gov/

This website offers information on a number of health conditions, including coronary artery disease, high cholesterol, angina, arrhythmia, atherosclerosis, and myocardial infarction (heart attack). It also provides descriptions of diagnostic tests, such as cardiac MRI and coronary calcium scanning. You can also learn about procedures, including cardiac catheterization, coronary artery bypass graft (CABG) surgery, and stenting.

DIETS

American Heart Association/American College of Cardiology Guidelines

www.heart.org/HEARTORG/HealthyLiving/HealthyEating/Healthy-Eating_UCM_001188_SubHomePage.jsp

Visit the Healthy Eating page on the AHA website for nutrition guidelines, tips on dining out, cooking videos, recipes, and tools to spot healthy foods at the grocery store.

USDA Food Patterns

www.cnpp.usda.gov/USDAFoodPatterns

Learn more about the USDA Food Patterns dietary guidelines, browse cookbooks, and watch cooking videos.

DASH Diet

http://dashdiet.org/

Discover more about the DASH diet and how to incorporate it into your daily life. This website includes links to DASH diet books available for purchase as well as dozens of free recipes you can start making now. You'll also find a section on FAQs to help you get started.

Mediterranean Diet

Because the Mediterranean diet is a style of eating rather than a specific diet, there isn't one catchall website for it. However, you can find a Mediterranean diet food pyramid at mediterradiet.org (just click on "The Pyramid" on the home page) and a meal plan and beginner's guide here (https://www.healthline.com/nutrition/mediterranean-diet-meal-plan#section7).

Plant-Based Diets

There are too many websites on vegetarian, vegan, and other plant-based diets to include here. To help you find the right plant-based diet for you, check out this article from Harvard Health Publishing (www.health.harvard.edu/staying-healthy/the-right-plant-based-diet-for-you).

SMOKING CESSATION

Smokefree.gov

https://smokefree.gov/

Created by the Tobacco Control Research Branch of the National Cancer Institute, this website offers information about a variety of topics related to quitting smoking, phone and text messaging support, and apps and other tools to help you stop smoking. You'll discover tools and tips to help you create a quitting plan, overcome the obstacles to quitting, and stay smoke-free for good.

GLOSSARY

Acute coronary syndrome (ACS): Cardiac events that are medical emergencies, including unstable angina and heart attack.

Angina: Angina pectoris, or simply angina, is chest pressure or pain that occurs when the heart doesn't receive enough oxygenated blood.

Angiogram: A coronary angiogram, which uses special X-ray imaging to see your heart's blood vessels, is considered the gold standard of diagnostic tests for detecting arterial blockages.

Angioplasty: A procedure that opens clogged arteries to improve blood flow to the heart.

Angiotensin: A chemical substance that narrows blood vessels, which increases blood pressure and forces the heart to work harder.

Angiotensin converting enzyme (ACE) inhibitors: Drugs prescribed to lower high blood pressure and to help heal the heart muscle after a heart attack. ACEs prevent the formation of angiotensin, which narrows blood vessels.

Angiotensin II receptor blockers (ARBs): Prescribed for high blood pressure, these drugs block the action of angiotensin. ARBs widen blood vessels to allow improved blood flow and lower blood pressure.

Antiarrhythmics: Medications that are prescribed to correct irregular heart rhythms, sometimes seen after a heart attack.

Anticoagulants: Drugs that thin the blood and prevent it from clotting.

Antiplatelets: Medications that prevent blood clots by inactivating platelets, the blood cells that help your blood form clots.

Aorta: The main coronary artery that directs blood from the heart to the rest of the body.

Arrhythmia: Irregular heart rhythms, such as atrial fibrillation, ventricular tachycardia, ventricular fibrillation, and bradycardia.

Artery: A blood vessel that carries blood from the heart to the body.

Atherosclerosis: The process that causes the inner wall of the coronary arteries to become damaged, narrowed, and clogged, leading to coronary heart disease.

Atria: The two chambers located at the top of the heart.

Atrial fibrillation: A type of arrhythmia in which the heart beats chaotically.

Beta blockers: Blood pressure medications that are also prescribed to alleviate chest pain. These drugs lower heart rate, allowing the heart to pump with less force, and widen blood vessels to improve blood flow and reduce blood pressure.

Biomarkers: Measurable substances in the body that indicate whether a person is experiencing ACS or heart attack.

Blood pressure: A measurement of the pressure created within your arteries as blood pumps through them. Blood pressure is expressed in two numbers—systolic (top number) and diastolic (bottom number)—and is given in millimeters of mercury (mmHg).

Bradycardia: An abnormal heart rhythm in which the heart beats too slowly.

Calcium channel blockers: Blood pressure medications often used to alleviate chest pain. They block calcium from entering the cells within the heart and in the blood vessels, relaxing the arteries and allowing blood to flow more freely to the heart muscle.

Cardiac catheterization: A procedure used to evaluate cardiac blood flow and heart function and to treat certain heart conditions.

Catheter: A long, thin, plastic tube that is threaded through an artery during cardiac procedures, such as angiography and stenting.

Cholesterol: A waxy substance that the body needs to build cells. Too much cholesterol in the blood is associated with an increased risk of CHD.

CK-MB: An isoenzyme that increases due to damage to the heart muscle. It is normally present only in trace amounts in the blood or may even be undetectable, but levels rise following a heart attack. In cases of ACS, levels of this isoenzyme are evaluated with a blood test.

Computed tomography angiogram (CTA): A minimally invasive diagnostic test that uses X-rays to examine blood flow in the coronary arteries.

Creatine kinase: An enzyme that plays a role in muscle function. In cases of ACS, a blood test is performed to determine whether levels of this enzyme are elevated, which indicates muscle damage and may point to a heart attack.

Coronary arteries: The blood vessels that take blood from the heart to the rest of the body.

Coronary artery bypass grafting (CABG) surgery: A surgical procedure in which blood vessels from the body are used to bypass blocked arteries.

Coronary heart disease (CHD): A condition in which coronary arteries are narrowed, increasing the risk of heart attack.

Coronary MRI: A minimally invasive diagnostic imaging test that uses magnets and radio waves to produce images of your heart.

C-reactive protein (CRP): High levels of this protein are associated with inflammation that indicates a higher risk of CHD.

Diabetes mellitus: A condition in which the body doesn't produce or doesn't respond adequately to the hormone insulin, resulting in abnormally high blood sugar levels.

Echocardiogram: A diagnostic test that uses ultrasound to create images of your heart as it beats and pumps blood.

Electrocardiogram (EKG): A diagnostic test used to evaluate the electrical activity of the heart.

Fibrinogen: A substance that contributes to blood clotting.

Heart attack: A heart attack occurs when one or more coronary arteries become clogged or narrowed, limiting blood supply to the heart and damaging heart tissue.

High blood pressure: Also called hypertension, this condition causes the heart to work harder and increases the risk of CHD.

High-density lipoprotein (HDL) cholesterol: This "good" type of cholesterol is considered to be protective against CHD.

Homocysteine: High levels of this amino acid found in the blood are associated with a risk of developing premature CHD and are linked to low levels of certain B vitamins.

Intra-aortic balloon pump: A mechanical device used to help the heart pump more blood.

Intravascular ultrasound: A diagnostic test that uses sound waves inside the blood vessels to evaluate the health of your coronary artery walls.

Left anterior descending (LAD) artery: Called "the widowmaker" because a blockage in this artery often results in death.

Lipoproteins: Proteins that transport cholesterol through the blood.

Lp(a): A type of lipoprotein that transports cholesterol, fats, and protein in the blood vessels. High levels of Lp(a) are associated with increased risk of CHD.

Low-density lipoprotein (LDL) cholesterol: This "bad" type of cholesterol is associated with a greater incidence of heart disease.

Metabolic syndrome: A cluster of medical conditions associated with increased chances of developing CHD.

Myocardial infarction: A medical term for a heart attack.

Myocardial perfusion imaging (MPI): A diagnostic test that uses a non-invasive scan to evaluate blood flow to the heart muscle.

Nitrates: Antianginal medicine that expands coronary arteries to relieve chest pain.

NSTEMI: A type of heart attack in which blood flow to the heart is limited but does not result in permanent damage to the heart muscle.

Nuclear stress test: A diagnostic test that involves taking two sets of images of the heart—at rest and during physical activity—to evaluate blood flow.

Optical coherence tomography (OCT): A diagnostic test that uses near-infrared light to produce high-resolution images of the blood vessels.

Plaque: Plaque is a buildup of cholesterol, calcium, and other substances in a coronary artery. Plaque can narrow arteries and contribute to a heart attack.

Platelets: Components in blood cells that promote clotting.

Silent ischemia: When blood flow to the heart is temporarily limited but does not produce any noticeable symptoms.

Statins: Medication used to lower cholesterol with an emphasis on reducing LDL levels.

STEMI: A type of heart attack that blocks blood flow to the heart and results in permanent damage to heart muscle tissue.

Stents: Narrow mesh tubes used to widen narrowed coronary arteries.

Stress test: A diagnostic test that involves walking on a treadmill or riding a stationary bike to evaluate heart function.

Sudden cardiac arrest: A devastating condition that causes the heart to stop beating and usually results in death.

Tachycardia: A type of arrhythmia in which the heart beats too fast.

Thrombolytics: Medicine used to break up clots in the bloodstream in cases of ACS and heart attack.

Thrombin: A substance that senses when there is damage to the inner wall of an artery and activates blood-clotting agents.

Thrombus: A platelet-rich blood clot.

Triglycerides: A type of fat in the blood that, when elevated, is associated with plaque formation and may increase the risk of CHD and heart attack.

Troponin: A protein in the blood that, when elevated, is a strong indicator of a heart attack.

Unstable angina: The acute onset of severe chest pain or prolonged chest pain that isn't associated with physical exertion and that elevates the risk of heart attack.

Vasodilators: A type of medication that reduces blood pressure by widening blood vessels.

Vein: A blood vessel that carries blood to the heart.

Ventricles: The two lower chambers of the heart.

Ventricular fibrillation: A dangerous type of arrhythmia in which the heart quivers rather than beating, leading to sudden cardiac arrest.

Ventricular tachycardia: A type of arrhythmia in which irregular electrical signals in the ventricles cause the heart to beat too quickly.

VLDL: A lipoprotein that transports cholesterol as well as triglycerides in the blood.

ACKNOWLEDGMENTS

The support and efforts of many people have helped make this book possible. I would like to offer my heartfelt thanks to my wonderful family for all the love and support they give me daily. I would also like to express my deepest gratitude to my staff, whose tireless efforts and dedication to our patients are greatly appreciated.

I would especially like to offer a hearty thank you to all the patients with whom I have been fortunate enough to meet. I am honored to care for you. I love hearing your stories, and I learn so much from every one of you. You motivate me to want to continue educating myself about heart health so I can provide you with the most advanced care so you can live your best life. You truly are the inspiration behind this book.

Finally, I would like to acknowledge Frances Sharpe for her invaluable editorial contributions in shaping this book.

INDEX

Type 1 diabetes. *See* diabetes mellitus
Type 2 diabetes, 140. *See also* diabetes
  mellitus
    insulin and, 29–30
    obesity and, 140
    trans fats and risk of, 125

U
unsaturated fats. *See* monounsaturated fats
  (MUFAs); polyunsaturated fats (PUFAs)
unstable angina, 15, 72, 92

V
vaping. *See* smoking
varenicline, 172–173
Vasotec, 81
vegan diet, 149
ventricles, 8
ventricular septal defect, 118
verapamil, 80
Verelan, 80
visceral fat, 140
vitamin B3, 87–88
VLDL (very low-density lipoprotein),
  23–24, 136

W
weight loss, 139–151. *See also* obesity
Welchol, 86
Wellbutrin, 173
widowmaker, 5–6

Z
Zestril, 81
Zetia, 87
Zocor, 85
Zyban, 173

Made in the USA
Lexington, KY
03 September 2018